HYPNODONTICS

Ethical Influence: Language for Dental Professionals

Juan P. Acosta, CHP

www.Hypnodontist.com

ISBN: 978-1-5003-1112-4
Published by Hypnodontist.com

This book carries a distribution license that allows professional hypnotists seeking to expand into the Hypnodontics market to have a great tool in their hands to help their local dental practices.

DISCLAIMER: The content of this book can help you make your dental patients more comfortable and your practice more profitable. However, we Juan P. Acosta/Hypnodontist/Its associates and affiliates, cannot guarantee the performance of your team. We do not make any income claims and we bring this volume to you with the intent to educate and enhance the quality of all the lives you touch, including yours. Your success with the skills taught in this book is directly proportional to the amount of time and effort you devote to practicing and growing, as you learn the language of ethical influence.

For more information about how hypnodontics can help please visit
www.Hypnodontist.com

Praise for Hypnodontics

"I am looking forward to applying the techniques in this book to help my patients. I believe "Hypnodontics" will add great value to my practice, where we strive to give optimal dental care with comfort and in a friendly environment. We'll do anything we can to make our patients more comfortable." **Isabel C. David, DDS. APC. Encinitas, CA**

"Without a doubt, this book can help every single dental office. Read it. Study it. Then reread it. It works." **Marvin Pantangco, DDS**

"It has been my experience that Juan Acosta is able to blend the art of clear communication with patient leadership to influence the patient's desire for dental excellence and willingness to pay for it. People do not "need" a smart phone, they want a smart phone. Juan transforms patients' "low level need" for dentistry into a "want" for it." **Evan Harris, Patterson Dental**

"As a clinical dental hygienist and hypnotherapist I am so thrilled Juan Acosta has written this book. His knowledge and use of "hypnotic language" in dentistry provides dental professionals the right practical tools to be more successful in all arenas of their work. Read it, apply it and watch your success unfold." **Jackie Foskett, RDH, C.Ht.**

To all who continuously stand behind me and push me forward, especially my Mother.

I'm so happy and grateful to have you.

TABLE OF CONTENTS

Foreword

In 2003 I began working as a hypnotist on staff in a dental practice. In the years since I have been fortunate enough to see for myself the variety of ways hypnosis and its principles can be employed in a dental office. I have met and worked alongside many dental professionals who have shared a positive outlook on dental hypnosis but don't have the resources to develop personal competency in the subject.

A few years ago I met Juan Acosta, a colleague passionate about helping connect hypnosis practitioners and dental professionals to improve patient outcomes as well as practice operations. His plan to educate and introduce both sides immediately made sense to me, as it allows all parties to share a common goal and language. His passion and skill-set will show themselves early in this book and readers will quickly see the excitement and logic he brings to this endeavor.

This book represents one of the initial major steps towards Juan's goal of facilitating a better relationship between dental and hypnosis professionals. I trust you'll take away from this book practical pieces you can incorporate with your patients immediately, and to see the potential for more with additional training and practice.

Scott Sandland, C.Ht.
Founder of the Hypnosis Practitioner Training Institute and Hypnothoughts.com (the largest hypnosis network on earth with over 16,000 members as of 2014)

Introduction

Dental anxiety and other unconscious behaviors are major contributors to poor oral health. Over the last two years I dedicated my time to bringing comfort to the dental practice in an effort to change that.

Having gone through specialized training for common mind/body dental issues like teeth grinding and TMJD, overactive gag reflex and insomnia, etc, I knew the dental field could use me, but at first I was shortsighted... I saw opportunities for patients to benefit from this approach and it gave me a great sense of satisfaction to help them, but I didn't realize the greater impact I could have on the rest of the dental practice's day to day operations.

In 2012 I had the opportunity to manage a dental clinic, and while working there my direct interaction with almost a thousand patients, several dozen doctors and other dental professionals helped me broaden how I view the scope of my work.

Suddenly I began to notice my skills were helping the practice grow due to reduced no shows, more and better online reviews and referrals, and increased patient satisfaction and retention. All that in addition to the already improved patient outcomes, faster healing times, and associated benefits of reducing chemical anesthesia and prescription drugs.

With a new outlook I began to work with other dental practices, and the scope of the trainings offered at Hypnodontist grew to include the language of ethical influence for dental professionals, which helps practices: increase case acceptance, revive old lists of patients who haven't scheduled, and generally finding ways for patients to elect to do the dentistry work their mouths need.

Within these pages then, dear dental professional, you will find effective communication techniques to help you become even more efficient and influential with your patients and other team members.

To put it simply, this book will help you offer your patients the type of complementary care that shows them how much you care, and it will teach you and your team how to keep them as patients and friends for life.

I applaud your dedication to your patients' experience, and trust we'll get to work together some time in the future.

Let's get moving!

Hypnodontics

Unwanted unconscious behaviors show up in all fields of health care. In dentistry, they present themselves in the form of fears and phobias, dental anxiety, overactive gag reflex, teeth grinding/clenching, insomnia, or undesired habits like smoking and nail biting, to name a few.

Hypnodontics deals with eliminating the symptoms of these conditions and in many cases the conditions themselves. Although "formal" hypnosis isn't used in any of the techniques in this book, you'll soon understand how "hypnosis" in a broader sense is the perfect addition to the excellent care you already provide.

Understanding the profound effect our words and actions can have on treatment outcomes makes the art of effective patient communications a skill worth learning. As a bonus when you apply them, the concepts and techniques you're about to learn will enhance every other area of your life.

Unlike other dental specialties, Hypnodontics deals only with the mental portion of your patients' oral health, not with the teeth themselves.

This Book

This book is about your developing a useful, practical skill-set which helps you make your patients comfortable and your practice more profitable. What you'll learn here will dramatically improve your patients' experience with you and your services, and thereby their quality of life and the sustainability of your practice.

There are 5 key elements in the paragraph above:

Development: As it's the case with any other skill worth learning, becoming proficient enough to be useful requires you understand the learning process.

Up until now you may have never thought of using hypnosis and the mind/body approach in your dental office. So up until now, it had been excusable for you to unknowingly miscommunicate with your patients, possibly asking them to experience more pain or anxiety than necessary... Yes, ignorance is bliss.

Now, after reading this volume with the intent to truly understand the subject, your new awareness will begin to turn the skills you will have learned here into unconscious competence, only as fast as you are able to practice and apply these skills with a live person. So practice practice practice. When the words flow easily and you catch yourself succeeding with these skills, then they'll have become second nature. Unconscious Competence.

Practical: What you'll learn in this book about hypnosis in dentistry are effective communication skills. Since we communicate in every interaction we have with another human, the skills are practical in any area of life where you want to apply them.

Useful: What if by reading this book and making a conscious effort to practice these skills, you were able to calm down a patient that is hysterical about having treatment done? Or to help a patient who is allergic to chemical anesthesia enjoy the same quality of oral care as other patients? Or to easily motivate a patient to comply with your requests to brush and floss regularly...? The usability of the information in this book is endless, and the more you learn about it, the easier it seems to find more applications for it.

So I encourage you to delve in as deeply as you want to be effective, having fun with the skills as you learn so that practicing will be effortless. If this is a chore for you, stop now. If this is fun for you, the rewards will be endless. You have my word.

Quality of life: Chances are one of the main reasons you entered the dental field was your desire to help others enjoy their experience of living, through better dental hygiene and oral health. This book will help you help more people, and you'll be able to help them in the most meaningful way... by taking the suffering out of their visit to the dentist. It is the suffering that hurts, not the pain. More about that later.

As a Hypnodontics trained dental professional you'll be much better prepared to help your patients improve the quality of their life. Think about it... There's only a small percentage of the population who doesn't mind going to the dentist, and nobody wants a toothache. When you're able to help patients relieve their pain and anxiety by talking to a patient in new and different ways, you'll be moving closer to your purpose.

Sustainability: Many practices struggle because they are missing pieces of the puzzle. Some are great at bringing new patients in for an inexpensive introductory appointment but they don't have a proper protocol for converting them into lifetime patients. Others get good case acceptance but have a difficult time keeping their hygienist busy.

The techniques and attitudes in this book and any Hypnodontist training are designed to help maximize your chair and production time, while increasing patient satisfaction.   A full chair + happy patients = Sustainability.

Practicing

Reading this book won't make you an expert. *Practicing* the skills you've read about will.

In my years of hypnosis and NLP (Neuro-Linguistic Programing) training, I have concluded the best way to internalize these skills so they become second nature is as follows. Take these steps with a little discipline and you will surely enjoy seeing yourself progress very quickly.

1. Read this book in its entirety once to understand the concepts and have a grasp of the scope of what you're learning. It's a short read and I expect it will become a book you refer to often.
2. After reading once, pick one concept that caught your attention. Maybe one that gave you the feeling of being useful for your practice right away.
3. Re-read the section dealing with that particular concept or skill and whatever related info that can help you make its application easier and more natural.
4. Spend a few minutes coming up with some specific situations in your life in which you could apply that skill, and decide how you will use it when it's time.
5. Practice that concept or skill EXCLUSIVELY for 3-5 days, and only move on to the new skill when you've had enough repetitions of "your lines" and they've

now become sort of automatic. No need to be perfect, just need to be teaching your unconscious mind the kind of responses you expect from now on.

When I started studying hypnosis I wanted to eat, drink, and sleep hypnosis. I was too fascinated to slow down and I wanted to get good at this now, not in a year or two... So in order to get exposure to enough people I could practice with, I went to work as a restaurant server. Where else can one have 2 to 6 or more captive people to "play with" in a setting where if a skill goes wrong the worst that can happen is they don't buy wine or dessert?

Your advantage of course is you already have a captive audience in your dental office, so there's no need to go get another job. There's only a need for you to give yourself permission to "mess up", understanding that learning is a process, and be willing to ease your skills into your daily life as you become more and more comfortable and proficient with them.

Every time they smile in amazement at what you've helped them discover or you catch yourself effortlessly using your new skills, your feelings of confidence and competence grow exponentially. Interestingly enough, as your confidence grows, so does your ability to influence your patients and listeners in a meaningful way.

Suggestibility & Belief

Humans are suggestible by nature. If I were to ask you to think about the process of going to your kitchen, looking through your silverware cabinet, taking a metal fork out of the drawer, and then biting it... chances are you've just had at least a minor physical reaction to a simple game of imagination.

What makes hypnosis work for millions of users worldwide is the fact that the human mind can create very real responses from imaginary events, if they are imagined vividly and with enough detail, as in the case of the metal fork example above where your body gets to experience a physical reaction from simply reading some words on a page and following a train of thought.

The good and the bad news... you're not alone. The people who come to your office for treatment are as suggestible as the rest of your team, the vendors and reps who visit you, and your family and friends. So the power of this information is strictly in its application.

Hypnosis then becomes the art of directing a person's suggestibility in the direction we want the person to **want** to act.

I'll let you digest that for a moment...

Yes, the hypnotic techniques you'll learn throughout this book will help you create change from the inside out.

In the coming chapters you will be trained and encouraged to speak as if your patients' outcomes depend on your communication, because largely they do!

Having dealt with several hundred dental patients looking for a caring listener it became evident to me that even though we're all people, we hold different beliefs and priorities and experience even the same experiences differently than the next person.

This has led me to believe... there's that word again... that all beliefs, no matter how strongly held by one person, could and do mean absolutely nothing to the next. So the managing of these beliefs is the first step in effective and efficient communications.

Pre-framing, Framing and Re-framing

The management of beliefs and expectations is an essential key in delivering on those expectations, which is where confirmation of the change occurs.

If the patient expects the needle to hurt because you told her it will... just a little... then it will. The problem is you have no idea if "just a little" for you might mean a whole lot of pain for the other person.

As with any human interaction, it's important to build rapport and be centered and empathetic. Being fully present will help position you as the authority and help patients relax, knowing they are in good hands.

In training, teaching and sales, it's commonly said you tell your listeners what you're about to tell them, then you tell them, and then you tell them what you've told them. This is similar.

Pre-framing is giving glimpses and clues of a successful outcome before the procedure takes place. I have been present in hundreds of surgeries and in almost every one of them (until they've trained with me) the team and doctors say things like:

- You're going to feel some pressure... there should be no pain though...

- Your face is a little swollen so the anesthetic won't work...
- Don't worry, if it still doesn't get numb, I will give you more…

If you read the section on suggestibility, you might understand why these are not Hypnodontist approved.

Whatever we focus our mind on, becomes our reality. As a quick example, if you just took a moment to notice that sensation on your feet…

you may begin to realize every breath you take... seems to make that sensation on your feet…

 a little more noticeable.

See, a moment ago your mind was focused elsewhere. Then I asked you about your feet and you were able to produce a physical sensation out of nowhere. So here are some better ways to create a response.

When you're about to give them a shot, say: "Most people feel pretty comfortable, but even if there's any pressure momentarily, they feel comfortable almost immediately after."

I know it seems like a simple phrase, but here's the breakdown of all the strings we're pulling with this phrase. It uses the principle of social proof, embedded commands, pacing and future pacing. It essentially tells the patient they should expect to feel almost nothing, but it also accounts for the fact that they could, because they are human. It also manages their expectations about what would happen if they did. It uses escape clauses like "usually" and "almost", and diminishes even the unlikely pressure to "if there's any."

You will learn some of these techniques and how to integrate them into your speech throughout this book.

When you know the anesthetic will need a little boost to create the same effect, you can say: "Since your face is swollen, we need to make sure the anesthetic will numb right here. Please concentrate on numbing that spot"

Since swollen faces can make it difficult for anesthesia to work, setting the patient's attention and intention on helping it work better, improves the outcome. More on boosting anesthesia in the "WANTED - Less Chemicals" section.

The phrase above also uses embedded commands, confusion, and ambiguity via vague language, which you will learn about in detail later.

So pre-framing refers to the set up work you do in preparing another person for something. You are setting the context for the communication you're about to send, to be received as planned.

Imagine a movie scene of a guy robbing a bank... pretty typical, right? Here are three of the endless possible pre-frames to illustrate my point:

1. Before the bank robbery scene, they show him preparing with a whole team of thieves for their final and biggest score ever. After the robbery they plan to retire on an exotic island and sip piña coladas from a coconut for the rest of their lives.

1. Before the bank robbery scene, they show him caring for his daughter as he kneels by her hospital bed and promises her that he will do anything to get the money for her operation.

1. Before the bank robbery scene, they show him as the terrorists wrap him up in explosives and force him to go into the bank and rob it.

How profound does the effect of pre-framing seem now?

If you only show the bank robbery itself... your viewer, listener, or patient, gets a version of your story that leaves a lot of room for interpretation. Pre-framing is the foundation of everything you will do (hypnotically) with your patients.

Once a frame of reference has been established (by you), it's important to keep it consistent throughout the rest of the interaction. When you set the frame you set an expectation that you must now deliver on. Sounds like a lot of work... but at least it's an expectation you know and understand. Nothing worse than working hard to deliver a top notch offering (of anything) only to find out the expectation of the recipient called for something completely different.

Framing then becomes a game of staying congruent with your suggestions and instructions, and always delivering a consistent attitude and intent. Consistent input creates change. It's simple conditioning.

Re-framing is a commonly used therapeutic tool. It shifts the focus of an interaction from its current less-than-ideal frame (expectation, context, belief or point of view) to a new frame that will be more useful going forward and more conducive to achieving the desired outcome.

To illustrate, let's say the scene of the man robbing the bank was the opening scene of the movie so there was no pre-frame. You watch the cold hearted robber order people around at gun-point, punch an old lady, lock the bank employees in the vault, and walk away with a large bag of cash... and then on the next scene he's freeing his family who was being held hostage and you learn that he was being forced to rob the bank to protect his family.

Maybe your perspective about what the guy is doing has shifted from where it started. Reframing is about finding the best possible perspective and offering it to the listener.

If you've ever said something like "well look at it this way" and then proceeded to explain how something could be understood differently if shown in a different context, you have already used re-framing in your communication.

Here's a dental example: A patient says "That implant is so expensive..." you can reframe it by saying "I realize that is a lot of money. I had a patient who was pretty concerned about that as well, but then he realized this is a fine custom made piece that will last him for the next 20 years and he said 'Wow... I guess that's a pretty good deal after all'. So if you look at it that way, I suppose having a great smile and the ability to eat normally for the next 20 years for only $3000 is not that bad. Is it?"

Ok, now take the "salesy" feel off the above example, and just understand the concept of reframing as offering a new perspective on something. We've all done it through life, naturally.

Building Rapport

Rapport is the connection we create with another human at a level outside of our conscious awareness. Our body language, attitude, speech, attire, mannerisms, etc. all play a role in our ability to connect with others.

Building good rapport is essential to our ability to influence. Under normal circumstances of course… The bank robber can be very persuasive with a gun and have no rapport.

It's commonly known that: people like people whom they perceive to be like themselves. It's the reason sales people ask fact finding questions to a prospect, so they can find some common ground to talk about, to build a relationship in which the prospect feels comfortable enough to buy.

Building rapport is the foreplay of communicating and influencing effectively. Here are some ways to do it:

Pacing & Leading

They say in order to lead someone out of the forest you can't just stay outside of it, calling their name… you must go in, find them, and show them the way out.

Pacing is the process of meeting a person wherever s/he is. So to pace, we can make a couple of comments about things we can observe which must be true for the patient. Then we can offer a leading suggestion.

Suggestions for patients to act upon are delivered precisely and deliberately, with your full intent on having the desired effect. That being said, they can be spoken as direct commands or blended into a story or metaphor to be interpreted by the patient via implied meaning. In the chapter on hypnotic communication you will learn more about delivering suggestions. For now, here's an example of this pace, pace, lead process in the dental office.

Say you're preparing a patient for treatment and you've given her an informed consent form to sign. While you prepare to anesthetize, the interaction could go something like this:

You: While you sit there, reading this consent, you can just relax for a moment. (pause) and now that you've signed, as I lean you back, you might imagine how great your smile will look in just a little while... (pause) leaning back now, looking up towards the light, allowing yourself to feel only comfort... and so on.

This pace, pace, lead pattern can be the basis for how you always deliver certain suggestions. What it can do for you is add predictability to your outcomes.

If you're always communicating with your patients with the same intent, to influence them to have appropriate responses to your suggestions, then you might begin to notice your percentages get better steadily.

NOTE: Learning the skills on these pages is a process. If you practice intelligently AND diligently, soon you'll be able to anticipate a reaction and come up with a response, with much less conscious involvement. And after that, it will easily become second nature.

Pacing allows you to seem to your patient as if you are in their world, having the same experience, and therefore someone who is able to lead the way.

Truisms and observable details and behaviors are great places to start pacing. If you've ever seen any material on sales techniques, you may be familiar with the concept of a "yes set" as a way to build "yes momentum" before asking the person for the sale. This is accomplished in a similar way when you pace, pace, lead.

Matching & Mirroring

An extension of pacing, matching and mirroring refers to the outside of conscious awareness mimicking of the person you're talking to, in order to build rapport.

Sounds complicated but it isn't. There are many things we can match about the person we're talking to which will begin to create that sense of connection.

Keeping the matching and mirroring outside of conscious awareness is about timing and practice. Paying attention to subtleties and details will yield great results.

The following are the building blocks of your ability to truly connect with your patient at a deeper level. The more of them you can match, the easier it will be to begin to lead in a new direction:

Posture: Our minds and bodies are connected so one affects the other. Do this exercise really quickly. I can appreciate the fact you're probably sitting down and relaxing as you read, but go ahead and stand up for just a moment.

Stand as straight as possible holding the book/tablet/phone in front of you so you can keep reading. Push your shoulders back and take a couple of nice, deep breaths. Hold your weight up in a position where your body feels open and strong...

and now while holding that posture... try to feel weak, meek, and lacking confidence. What, you can't!?!? Probably not without sizable effort and even if you could, it would likely only happen with a change in your physical posture.

So if our body can dictate how our mind feels and vice-versa, how can you begin to put what you're learning here to good use?

An example of the dental application of pacing and leading by matching posture would be in talking to a very anxious person, who may be very closed in and protected, slouching and with their arms bent up as if guarding her heart.

One could approach that person with a similar posture and a subdued attitude, and slowly begin to open up to a more relaxed posture as rapport increases. Once the person's physiology opens up more it will be easier for her to accept any suggestions of wellbeing and comfort.

Sound: There are many elements of a person's voice that can be matched: Tone, Speed, Pauses, Intonation, Sounds they make...

If you think about a person's voice as the outward representation of what they're thinking, then exercising flexibility and easing yourself into the same patterns they use will help you communicate with their thoughts. Kind of creepy... but it's true.

Language: The words, accents and sayings your patients use already hold an emotional meaning for them.

Listening to their language choices, you can learn what works for them and effectively influence them in a way that is already part of their natural process.

People will use words repeatedly or with a certain emphasis which gives us clues about their preference towards them. The key words you want to pace are the ones the patient uses to describe things. Those are words with an emotional component attached to them.

Here's an example of a patient interaction in which the patient's language preferences are paced and then the conversation is lead to begin to relieve pain.

Pt: I have a TERRIBLE toothache, I haven't been able to sleep for 3 days because of it and it's making me MISERABLE.

You: Ouch, I'm sorry. I know toothaches can make people really **miserable**. Let me ask you, is the pain always **terrible** or does it get better or worse when you chew or drink?

Pt: Well, it's constantly there but it gets a lot worse when I drink anything cold or bite on that side.

You: Oh, I understand. So it's terrible when you bite or drink, but lighter when you're just sitting there... (patient nods in agreement) Ok. And are there some things that make it feel better?

Pt: Yeah, Oragel makes it feel AWESOME, but only for a little while.

You: Ok, **awesome**. Well let me put some of this topical anesthetic on it to get you nice and comfortable while I come back. It's like doctors' strength Oragel so you should feel **awesome** in just a moment.

And so on...

Essentially, you're meeting the patient where they are feeling miserable with a terrible toothache, and gradually guiding them into a more awesome state of mind in which they are feeling comfortable and preparing for treatment.

The above example is simple and straight forward but you can make this process as fancy and intricate as you'd like. The amount of playfulness you apply to these techniques is directly proportional to how well they will work. The most important skill to learn here is listening.

Movement: Similar to the language we use, humans have movements and mannerisms that characterize us.

You can pay specifically close attention to the movements your patients use when telling you those emotionally charged words like: terrible, miserable or awesome in the example above.

Using the same gestures patients use when you respond to them will let them know you've been listening (even if at a subconscious level), and help strengthen your connection so you can resolve their problem.

While it's true you don't want to use the same gestures immediately after the patient to minimize the risk of being caught mimicking them, you can allow your eyesight to de-focus so your peripheral vision takes over, and then slow down your "mimicking" response by a few seconds. This allows you to notice certain movements and even a person's breathing, without seeming as if you're fixated on them or planning something, and keeps the conversation flowing naturally.

Breathing: One of the most powerful yet undetectable techniques is to pace a person's breathing. By using your peripheral vision as explained above, you can begin to notice even small details in movement happening outside of your main field of vision.

A person's breathing rate dictates a lot of things, most importantly how fast they talk and when. By matching their breathing you can talk when they are exhaling as people normally do, which gives a moment of silence during the inhale to digest the previous thoughts and get ready for the next.

Our breath is tied to our emotions. Taking long deep breaths is naturally relaxing, while hyperventilating naturally causes an anxious response. So you can find an anxious patient where she is by pacing her breathing, and then lead into a better place.

Demeanor: Mismatching a person's demeanor is generally a bad idea. Think about what happens when someone is freaking out, yelling and making big arm and hand movements, very visibly agitated... If you're trying to talk sense into that person you may think you're doing the right thing by very calmly saying: Hey, just relax, it will be better soon... or whatever to that effect.

But the reality is those two demeanors are too far apart. Here again, you must go into the forest to lead the person out. A more appropriate response would be to match their movement, tone of voice and general demeanor, before gradually helping them into a better state.

Facial Expressions: Humans are so expressive... aren't we? Do this simple exercise.

- Go to the bathroom and look in the mirror

- Cover your mouth as much as possible from view but leave some space between your hand and your face so you can still talk and move your lips
- While looking at your eyes only, smile. A real smile...

Now...

Did you notice any changes in your eyes, eyebrows, nose, forehead, etc. when you smiled, that let you know you were smiling without having to actually see your smile?

I trust your answer is yes...

Facial expressions mean a lot to us and pacing them can create a deep sense of understanding and connection. Use them to your advantage.

5 Senses

Part of the uniqueness of being human, is how each of us chooses to represent the world we live in. And by it being a choice, I don't mean it's a conscious one.

If you've ever heard someone say they're very visual or so and so is touchy feely, you may already realize the importance people give to one or more of their senses.

Understanding your patients' preferred sense(s), or what in NLP we call "representational systems", gives you an edge when communicating with them. Think of these systems as different languages people use to express themselves... if you want the most direct line of communication you'll want to speak the same language.

The good news is we can all naturally communicate in all these languages. We just need to train ourselves to listen first, and then flip an imaginary switch that translates what we want to say into their preferred language or system, before we actually speak. How do we do that? We practice listening. A lot.

When people speak, clues in their language reveal their preferred system. For example a person who is very visual may say things like "I see what you mean" or "I hadn't looked at it that way". A person whose auditory sense is strongest may be heard saying "I hear you loud and clear" or "Oh yeah, that rings a bell". And you can connect with the kinesthetic person with "I feel your pain" or "I sense how difficult this is for you"

Generally when these systems are discussed, trainers stop at these three: visual, auditory and kinesthetic, because they are the most prevalent. However, in the dental field we do get the rare opportunity to work with taste and smell a little more than other professions.

Although the majority of the population will fall in the VAK categories, you can still pace the Olfactory and Gustatory senses since there are so many flavors and smells associated with being in the dentist's chair, and involving more of the senses creates what is known as synesthesia. A mixing of senses which allows for a feeling to have a color or a sound to have texture, etc.

Synesthesia can be elicited easily by mentioning the association you want to make. For example if I asked you about an experience you've enjoyed in the recent past and I said: Thinking about your recent experience... as you put yourself in that moment once again... seeing what you saw, hearing what you heard, and feeling what you felt... then you can let that enjoyable feeling grow inside. And if you could imagine that feeling inside being made of a colored vapor, so that as the feeling moves around you could see the streaks of where it's been and where it's going... now notice that the thicker the colored vapor gets... the stronger the feelings and the more intense the color becomes, the better it feels..."

Essentially we're encouraging the person we're talking to to get more of their senses involved. Why? Think of it this way:

How about such an intense experience as a roller coaster ride... in which you not only feel the movement of the car you're in, but you can also hear the clanking of the chain as the car slowly creeps up to the top... and then you might also remember how different things look as the roller coaster goes up and up and everything below, and the city around you seems to become smaller and smaller. As you look at the people around you, there are lots of smiles and a few faces of sheer terror as the ride nears the point of no return... who are we kidding, the point of no return was back in line... and as the ride goes over the top there's always that release of the chain; the ultimate "Clank" that let's you know the real fun is about to start... followed by a scream of released excitement by most people... and a prayer by a few others. And then, that sense of weightlessness takes over for a moment as the car drops down and the clanking of the chain is replaced with the exciting sound of the ride speeding on its rails...

I know it's a simplistic example. But in the paragraph above as you cycle through your senses by following the thoughts I'm giving you, you create within you a sensory overload much more intense than any one sense alone could give you.

Creating synesthesia gives people something extra to think about when they are experiencing pain or anxiety. Here's an example of something you could say to a patient to create synesthesia, and help them be in control of their own sensation as they go through a dental procedure:

"Alright Mr. Patient, let's get you nice and comfortable now. What I need you to do is notice when that sensation on your feet starts to become a little stronger... that's your sign that very soon you'll be numb enough to start the treatment. My patients say it makes it work better when they pay attention to what that sensation would sound like if it had a sound... or imagine it's a certain color so they can see it... (Then you anesthetize) ... Let me know when you're ready."

Here is a list with some sample words in the three main representational systems to get you started:

Visual	Auditory	Kinesthetic
Bright	Say	Attack
Appear	Sound	Catch
Look	Talk	Connect
Perspective	Tell	Tender
Picture	Speech	Touch
Watch	Hear	Solid
View	Harmony	Pressure
Ugly	Noise	Sense
Pretty	Quiet	Hurt
Show	Lecture	Grab
See	Call	Grasp
Glow	Discuss	Feel
Brilliant	Conversation	Firm
Glance	Describe	Point
Glare	Listen	Manipulate
Light	Speak	Hard
Envision	Tone	Rough
Dim	Tune	Push
Visible	Voice	Stable

More about the language used and some of the tongue-fu tricks above will be explained in detail as you move through the sections in this book. For now, let's get back to building rapport.

Identification

I like to tell the story about a day when I was driving through Pacific Beach, and at a stop light having my windows down and looking at what was going on around me, I noticed a mail man as he parked on my right side, got out of his car and grabbed a tub of people's mail.

As I waited for the light and watched the mail man put the tub down, right in front of the mail boxes, I began to imagine what it would be like to be him. Having to look at everyone's name and address, and finding the corresponding box for each envelope or package.

Then I got an even more interesting feeling as I thought about what the rest of the mailman's day would be like... waking up in the morning, spending a little time with his wife and kids... getting ready for work... and so on.

Imagining what it would be like if I were in his shoes, gave me a strange sense of connection with this person whom I'd never met or talked to. Had we had a chance to meet, the rapport between us would have built really fast, because I would have greeted him with a sense of empathy and a sense of understanding about him and his life.

This works with your patients because identifying with them like I did with the mailman, will help you connect with them to a level where they can feel you truly understand their experience.

You may have already noticed not one of these rapport building points works alone. An important thing to understand about hypnotic communication and rapport building is even though all these techniques are used by us naturally, until we have a conscious awareness of how we do what we do we'll continue to get unpredictable results.

Again, predictable results require practice. Lots of it.

Another current example is my ability to identify with you since I've been where you are right now... working up an appetite for these skills, and starting to get a sense of how broad a body of work this is. Looking forward through this book's table of contents it's easy to imagine how profound a transformation you'll have experienced in your ability to communicate effectively with your patients, when you have finished the book and have moved on to the practicing phase of your learning.

In fact, I'm willing to bet you can also identify with me... if you were to only think about how it would feel... to be able to use these skills in a flowing way in natural conversation, and having to decide what parts of this large body of work can be trimmed so it's an easy to digest volume, and not a brick... yet knowing there are still endless amounts of things to learn, and more being developed every day!

Whew... now that we know each other better... let's move on to one of best rapport building techniques available. And it's free!

Humor

A witty comment, a funny response, a humorous situation, even a joke, can relax the mood and open doors to communication.

Laughter creates a bond amongst people and it also offers natural pain relief, by promoting the release of endorphins, oxytocin, and other feel-good chemicals in the brain. Because our mind/body connection is so incredibly strong, this happens even when we force ourselves to laugh. The benefits of laughter are many.

While managing the dental clinic many times I suggested patients watch a funny movie or do something that would get them laughing between our call and their scheduled appointment time.

The Consequence of Thought

Human action is rooted in thought. Therefore if you want to learn how to move yourself and others to action, you must understand the relationship between thoughts, feelings, actions and results.

I'm sure you're familiar with the idea that when we make a purchase (or a decision), we do it based not on logic, but on emotion. When we have a thought... a memory... an idea... as it's interpreted in our brain it evokes certain emotions and feelings inside of us.

Those feelings prompt us to take action. What kind of action depends on what kind of feeling... and the actions we take and choices we make, ultimately create our results.

What should I say?

So this is all great. You understand that our thoughts directly or indirectly affect the results we achieve or don't achieve. And whether the action you're going after is for the patient to brush more often, or to achieve hypnotic anesthesia, the process works the same way.

While you become proficient with these skills, sometimes it's easy to get tongue tied and not know what to say next. Knowing what you now know, that will no longer be an issue for you. Here's why:

Your job as a facilitator is not to figure out what to say but to inspire thoughts that create the right type of feeling, that prompts people to take action in the direction of what they want or need. In the sections that follow, you'll learn how to turn your "what to say next?" question, into a "what feeling do I want to evoke?" question, and how to direct your listeners' attention where it needs to be to do that.

Are you ready? The next section starts the meat of the training you've been patiently waiting on, which is how to *actually* communicate to achieve the desired response.

By the way, if you want your team to be able to see and hear how this style of communication is supposed to be used, and learn more of the specific "what words to say" I encourage you to check out The Morning Huddle, the Hypnodontist recorded video training program where we teach your team the language of ethical influence so they can make your patients more comfortable and your practice more profitable.

Free training > http://Hypnodontist.com/tmh

For now, continue to enjoy the reading!

The Direction of Motivation

I always find it interesting when my clients tell me they don't have the motivation to do something. That if only they were more motivated their productivity would increase, they would become financially stable, they would have the time-freedom they want, blah blah blah...

What is actually happening is not that they don't have the motivation, because we all have that. It's that they don't understand the direction of their motivation. That's right, there is more than one type of motivation. Figuring out how your patients prefer to be motivated is the first step in structuring your communication to them for the best possible response.

The good news is it's easy, the bad news is the direction of a person's motivation can be situationally dependent.

For example, people can be motivated towards a goal or desire such as having a beautiful smile, or they can be motivated away from something such as in the case of a toothache or other ailment.

Towards: This type of motivation is generally regarded as the best type to have, because our brain does such as great job with details that it cannot distinguish the difference between a real experience and one that is vividly imagined. So having a towards motivation means when we motivate ourselves, we are rehearsing success, as opposed to rehearsing "not failure" - An important distinction.

Away: In my office, I teach my "away" motivated clients the pros and cons of their preference. In your dental office you won't need to do that. You simply need an understanding of that preference so you can influence your patient with less effort. A person motivated away from things doesn't get the benefit of rehearsing success... but it does make it easy to use techniques such as aversion.

Would you like to know the secret to quickly finding out the person's motivation strategy and lead them in the way they want to be led? Of course you do. Here it is:

Ask good questions, and listen.

In the same way people reveal their language choice being either Visual, Auditory or Kinesthetic, they reveal their motivation strategy. As the facilitator, your mission (should you wish to accept it) is to ask open ended questions which get the patients talking. An open ended question is one that requires an actual response, different than yes or no. Here are some ideas:

  - Ideally what would you like to happen?

- What are the main reasons why you want to deal with this now?
- If I could snap my fingers and grant you a wish regarding your oral health, what would that wish be?

The answers to these and other questions you can come up with, relevant to your own needs, may sound something like this:

- I just want to have healthy teeth
- I'd like to have a beautiful smile again
- I can't wait till I can eat again. Haven't eaten in days.
- I haven't been able to eat in days. I need to get rid of this pain
- I just want to take care of this before my insurance lapses
- I've had the toothache for months but now it got bad enough

Common responses like these are full of clues about how to motivate your patients. If you examine the answers above, you'll notice whether the patient is looking forward to something, or focused on what she doesn't want. Knowing that, tells you what buttons to push to get the patient in motion.

Incidentally, when I talk about getting the patient in motion, I'm referring to your ability to influence them to act in their best interest of course.

Understanding the direction of motivation can boost your effectiveness when: a) presenting a case, b) pushing for what you know is their best option if they're reluctant, c) asking them to adhere to your instructions to not smoke, brush and floss, etc. d) communicating with other team members in your office, etc.

Once you've learned their motivation style, you can begin to communicate with them using their preference. This makes them feel like you understand and care for them. Your responses then, could be:

- Great. If you want to have a healthy mouth, here's what I'd recommend
- Ok. The ceramic implant is going to give you the best smile
- I understand. So let's take care of your mouth before that insurance goes away
- No worries, in just a few hours you'll be able to eat again
- That's awful. I will get you out of here soon so you can take care of that hunger
- And so on...

When they reveal their motivation strategy, for the most part they don't know it. In essence, what you want to do is pace their strategy so they feel heard, and then you lead them onto the next step: Buying, making a decision, brushing their teeth, coming back next week, etc.

Subconscious Communication

There's talking... and then there's hypnotic communication. Meaning communication that isn't only words but more a direction of your listener's suggestibility by having: first the right attitude, and second, the right words. The right attitude you'll develop as you practice and learn. The "what to say" you're learning in this book.

Wordswordswordswords...

"I have a dream!" - How powerful can words be? - In your dental office your aim is not to influence the human race, but that doesn't mean that your words are any less important. To the patient in the chair, your words can mean the world. So when you're giving them the world, apply the golden rule and decide what kind of world you'd want them to experience.

Words can be swords. If thrown around carelessly they can dig deep and cause a world of pain and suffering. Hypnotic communication is about learning what words to use when, with what person; as well as what not to say.

Take these two examples of a patient in the dental chair, listening to their dentist say:

- Now I'm going to give you a shot, and don't worry about the pain, it hardly ever hurts, it's usually just pressure. But if it does, lift your left hand to let me know and I'll give you more... (give shot)

- Now I'm going to get you comfortable for the duration of your visit. People usually notice a different sensation on your feet, that lets us know it's working already. Signal when you feel it... (give shot)

Now ask yourself this: If you were the patient listening to the first spiel about the shot, what does that sentence get your mind focused on?

If you answered "pain" or "hurt" you are right. And what we focus on increases. So while you may have thought (before reading this) you were being helpful by telling the patient not to worry, etc. in reality those were just good intentions matched up to the wrong words.

The second phrase, by contrast, focuses the patient's attention as far away from the actual shot as possible (the feet) and asks them to notice the sensation, which will mean the anesthetic is working. The phrase is laden with language "tricks" which you'll learn throughout this book.

To recap, in the first example they're focused on: I need to lift my hand when it hurts. Keeping them searching for the pain so they can comply with your instructions. In the second, they're focused on: When I feel that sensation it will mean the anesthetic is working. And they'll always feel that sensation if you suggest it.

Don't believe me? Maybe it's because until now you weren't aware of that feeling on your hands... but now that you are... it should be easy to believe your patients will feel it too.

Keep the two examples above in mind, it will be useful to refer back to them as we move through the next several headings.

Process Language

This refers to the two different ways in which we can convey information. We can offer information to be received intellectually as in the case of a textbook, or experientially as in the case of much of this book, a movie, or a metaphor or story.

Process language conveys information in a way that the actual experience becomes the lesson. It provides a deeper understanding of whatever is said, because of synesthesia... (explained in the rapport building section.)

Here's an example of the difference between process language and the intellectual knowledge:

You could tell a patient she should relax and expect her to figure out how, OR... you could tell a patient to imagine herself enjoying some relaxing down time, doing whatever she loves. Essentially nudging a new thought pattern with relaxation as the goal. The process option invariably leads to better results, as simple as it is.

Artfully Vague

Milton H. Erickson, MD is considered to be the father of modern hypnotherapy. His approach in working with clients was to assist them to find resources within themselves by using thought provoking processes through natural conversation.

Being "artfully vague" means to offer open ended notions guided towards achieving the clients goals and letting the listener fill in the blanks for what could be, instead of giving them direct suggestions for change.

When a person feels as if they have found the knowledge on their own, as opposed to it being imparted upon them, change happens more rapidly and with less effort.

Think about it... we rarely reject our own ideas and they usually seem pretty good to us even if others think they're crazy. I experience this regularly! Haha.

Going back to the second phrase about the shot (above), you may notice we don't tell the patient WHAT sensation to feel, we simply say "a different sensation". That way if the patient is feeling tingling, or heaviness, or a change in temperature, they can all be correct. And whatever fits the patient's experience is what will make sense for them and ultimately ratify the changes taking place.

One could talk about: Those changes you want to make, That feeling on your hand, or the way it feels when you X.

All these sentences have an element of vagueness that sends the patient's mind into a search for meaning... In order for them to experience that feeling, they must first decide what that feeling is. This thought pattern creates what some people call trance, and increases their emotional investment in their results. The more they invest, the better results they'll achieve.

Affirmatively Speaking

Our mind is always on. In order for us to not think of something, we must first think of it and then delete it.

I know it sounds ridiculous... but consider this... what happens when I ask you to make sure you don't think about Sponge Bob, the cartoon...?

I hope you didn't think of it... did you? - Of course you did. At the very least you must have made a quick scan of the words "Sponge Bob" to see whether or not they have meaning for you, before letting your mind go elsewhere. In doing that, you made a representation (thought) of it.

Here's how can this be applied in your dental office. Again, it's all about focus:

Instead of saying	Say
you won't feel pain	you'll feel only comfort
this won't hurt	you'll feel almost nothing
don't worry	you're in excellent hands
try not to flinch	just stay relaxed
anything with "not" in it	an action in the affirmative

Language Patterns

Language patterns are collections of words strung together to create a result or a thought structure for your patients to follow. Their value is in eliciting the right thought process in their mind so you can begin to ethically influence the right emotions to get them to take action towards their/your desired outcome.

In this book, I will touch on some concepts for you to start creating your own patterns, but I highly recommend you study and practice language patterns by using tools like our Hypnodontist Morning Huddle video training or the "language cards" at saladseminars.com.

In the rest of this section I will share with you the concept behind language patterns, and also ways to ease them into conversation.

Embedded Commands (Action Steps)

What exactly is a command? It's a direct, authoritative request. In the case of subconscious communication, commands can be embedded in the things we say and go consciously unnoticed yet still carried out.

When you learn to embed commands or "action steps" you can more easily control the flow of communication. And as you practice these skills more and more, you may find yourself embedding action steps automatically, when you want to influence your patients, or become a better communicator.

Think about the way a "command" is delivered. I could, in an even and matter-of-fact tone, tell you to "practice these skills" because you must. Or... I could do it like I did in the paragraph above, where embedded the same action step by using the proper verb tense and presuppositions which you will learn about in the next section.

Look at the paragraph again and notice the phrases: Learn to embed commands; practice these skills; find yourself embedding action steps; want to influence your patients; become a better communicator.

When you first read them, you may or may not have noticed they were motivating words "selling you" on the fact you should learn these skills...

Ok, let's play. Take this last sentence as an example of how to construct a sentence for maximum impact. Here's the original phrase:

"'selling you' on the fact you should learn these skills"

I could have written:

"selling you" on learning these skills
"selling you" on becoming proficient at this
"selling you" on the benefits of understanding commands

But none of those choices have the proper verb tense for being delivered as a command. Instead of the present participle of the verb, meaning the ING ending, the command must be in it's infinitive form, meaning its most basic form which could have the word "to" in front of it, although it's not used in the action step itself. So the verbs of the examples above would have to change:

from "learning these skills" to "learn these skills"
from "becoming proficient at this" to "become proficient at this"
from "understanding commands" to "understand commands"

That's why I chose the phrase I chose. It leans on a "fact" (whatever that means) and urges you to "learn these skills"... in-fact, it tells you "you should!"

As you have now reread the above you may have felt an interesting sense like: Hmm... I can't believe all those commands were so blatantly written there and it just seemed like normal writing. That leads me to believe even more important than the command itself, is how to deliver it without becoming annoying or actually seeming authoritative. The answer is in presuppositions and assumptions.

Presuppositions & Assumptions

Are you familiar with the concept of assuming the sale? It means to go into a sales situation already acting as if the sale has taken place and thereby taking the focus away from the tension of "the sale" and moving onto the details. An example is when you're buying a car and the sales person asks: Will you be taking the red one or the more sporty blue one? Whichever you answer is only strengthening the position of the sales person.

Let's put presuppositions in the right context of how we use them to deliver commands by looking at the sample paragraph again:

The paragraph reads: **"When you <u>learn to embed commands</u> or "action steps" you can more easily <u>control the flow of communication</u>. And as you <u>practice these skills</u> more and more, you may <u>find yourself embedding action steps automatically</u>, when you <u>want to influence your patients</u>, or <u>become a better communicator.</u>"**

Notice all the underlined commands are delivered by an assumption of some sort...

"when you <u>learn to embed commands</u>" presupposes you are going to learn and it only leaves room for the right timing. Most importantly, it opens the door for me to use the proper verb tense and create the acton step.

And after all, it's not entirely about whether or not you want to control the flow of communication, but about how you can control it **"more easily."**

Also, **"As you <u>practice these skills</u>" "you may <u>find yourself embedding commands automatically</u>".** I don't know about you, but I'm curious about what would happen if you actually practice these skills as much as I'm encouraging you to…! It becomes a fun game and your patients will love you for it.

Of course you only have to practice this **"when you <u>want to influence your patients</u>, or <u>become a better communicator</u>"**… which I'm sure is only all the time.

Now let's go dental and examine the sample patter below for commands promoting relaxation. These can be: get/be comfortable, relax, etc. This little bit of patter we're about to dissect will be worth many times your investment in this book… if you USE IT in your practice!

If you were talking to a patient coming for treatment, as you lead him/her to the chair and build rapport, you could say something like this:

You: Okay _____, why don't you **take a load off… hear…** and **get comfortable.**

Pt: Thank you.

You: If there's anything else I can do to help you **relax even more** just let me know. While the hygienist/ doctor comes in, let's put a little of this topical anesthetic on so you can **be comfortable starting now**… no sense waiting, right…?

Pt: Haha, no. The sooner the better!

You: I know what you mean. Well, people usually **feel this topical anesthetic immediately.** When it touches you'll **feel that change in temperature** and that's how you **know it's working already**.

Pt: Oh yeah, that's really fast.

You: Great. Please tell me when you begin to **feel that comfort all the way down in your toes.** For some people it's almost instant, for others it takes a few seconds... Okay? ... I'll be right back.

Pt: Okay.

When you get back, your patient will have been focused on finding that relaxation while you were gone, and in doing so s/he can't help but feel it.

Using presuppositions to turn those action steps into their usable form we can expect to see more actions be consistent with our efforts.

Confusion & Ambiguity

For the same reasons and sometimes in conjunction with being artfully vague, confusion and ambiguous meanings send the patient's mind in a search for answers.

Suggestibility is enhanced when we are confused because in that (sometimes very brief) moment, the human mind will go for the low hanging fruit, as long as the low hanging fruit makes some sort of sense.

Meaning in a moment of confusion, our direct suggestions can be much more quickly acted upon.

Ambiguity is a great way to create that state of confusion and suggestibility. For example, I could ask you to think about the last time you had a choice to make... and just like when you are driving along a road and you get to a fork on the road, you could take the right path, or decide to take the path that's left. Because whether the left path is right or the right path is wrong, choosing is a right we all have, and the left path is actually the right choice. And while it's true many times it's impossible to know whether you've made the right choice, or taken the right path, you'll soon find out just how good a choice you were left with because that feeling will come along, and right away it can become clear the right choice was all that was left. I get a sense that right and wrong are both on the same path.

Now, if you're left thoroughly confused, that is absolutely right. Let's move on to a quick explanation.

In this very obvious example of ambiguity to create confusion, you may notice even though it all makes sense if you spend some time on it, as you read over it just once, it's difficult to keep track of what's going on because our brain is really busy, trying to decide which meaning of right or left is being used in which instance. The minor overload is what makes us reach for the easiest answer. I wonder what path you would take on the example above?

Confusion is the preceding state to learning. And since ambiguities create confusion then we can use them to install knowledge.

Let's look at how this can be accomplished by referencing two of the sentences used in the dental example above:

"take a load off... hear... and **get comfortable"** - Any time you have a chance to use an ambiguity, you have an opportunity to send the listeners mind into a quick search for meaning: Did he say hear? But surely he meant "here"... what, get comfortable? oh sure, THAT sounds good and that I can understand... and so the action step to "get comfortable" is more easily accepted and acted upon.

"no sense waiting" - What? Is there no sense in waiting to be comfortable... or is there such a thing as "no sense" just waiting to happen when the topical anesthetic begins to work?

In any case, confusion opens the door to suggestion. In the next section we'll discuss how to use tag questions to intensify the suggestions you've made and get a commitment from the patient to act accordingly.

Tag Questions

These quick questions confirm a statement that was just spoken. And golly, they're hard to disagree with. Aren't they?

Just think about the last time a tag question was used in your daily life. Surely you can remember at least one instance, can't you? - If you can't, just read the two sentences above for examples, and also the commitment we got from your patient above: "no sense waiting, right...?"

You see, questions that end a sentence after a statement is made, essentially "tagging" the sentence, make it easier for people to agree with the statement itself.

I think this is all the explanation tag questions need. Don't you?

It's easy to start using them with your patients and they make it easy to get them to create commitments like the one to be more comfortable sooner. But I'm sure you'll play with these and soon you'll see how effective they can be. Won't you?

Yeses

The word yes and other positive responses to your questions can begin to create an air of agreement and therefore promote collaboration from your listener. For example, you can just tell someone to go sit on the chair and relax, and that may work for some people. Or you can create smooth "yes momentum" so when you slip in the suggestion to "be comfortable" or "relax" it can be understood at a deeper level. Here's an example:

You: Alright _____, have a seat... beautiful day out there huh!? (they will agree... unless it isn't... and you'll continue) Is that comfy? (talking about the chair... most dentists' chairs are, so they will agree... and you'll continue) I bet you're ready to get this over with... (they will most likely agree... and then, having created a frame of agreement or "yes momentum" you can now add a direct suggestion or command) good, well just sit there and **get more comfortable by the minute** and the doctor will see you when **you're ready for this.**

These "yes sets", as they are commonly known as the oldest trick in the book for a sales person, put to work the concept of pacing and leading better than most other techniques. If you notice, in the example above we play a simple game of mentioning things that we already know the answer to... so we're purposely asking questions common to their experience in order to get them saying yes and feeling agreeable.

Little bits of common knowledge such as: I bet you're ready to get this over with; a shared experience such as: Beautiful day out there; or any other observable and simple bits of conversation you can come up with, are great pacing points.

Let's look now at the leading suggestion at the end of our yes set above: "good, well just sit there and **get more comfortable by the minute** and the doctor will see you when **you're ready for this**."

As you can see, the command doesn't ask them to find comfort… it presupposes comfort is already there by asking them to become "more" comfortable. It also adds a new timing clause. Riddle me this: If they're getting more comfortable by the minute… what will happen in 3, 5 or 10 minutes? That endless loop is created, helping them automatically and intensifying their experience of relaxation and comfort exponentially.

Lastly, we finish the suggestion above by quickly binding them (without their knowledge) by saying that when the doctor sees them, they'll be ready for this. And also notice that the suggestion is given in the form of an embedded command. The verb tense is strong, you're confidently nodding as you deliver it, and it gives the patient that extra little boost they needed to give themselves permission to relax.

I should mention that your delivery is just as important or more, than the words themselves. Body language, proper pausing, the right emphasis, and more, play an important role in the effectiveness of your suggestions. And THAT is the #1 reason for practicing until it becomes something you just do.

Buts

The patient would love to have a beautiful set of teeth, but she's deathly afraid of the dentist.

Based on only that information... do you think THAT patient will achieve her goal of a beautiful set of teeth?

The answer is no, unless there's a shift in her thinking. And that's where you come in. If you re-read that sentence you'll notice that at the beginning, the patient is motivated by a beautiful set of teeth. But then something changes... a condition... a hurdle, challenge, problem that stops her from having it. And the secret is all in the "but."

The word "but" effectively negates what was just said and redirects the attention to where it's most needed. The motivation.

I'm sure in your lifetime you've heard someone say to someone else: Hey, I love you BUT... followed by any number of remarks about that diminish the effect of "I love you" to the point where it's non-existent.

Knowing this gives us the ability to REVERSE the effect, by restructuring our communication and putting our buts in the right place. Follow this example and you'll get the gist of it in no time.

You: Hi (Pt. Name), how are you feeling?

Pt: Well I'm happy to get this fixed **but** I am so nervous.

You: I can appreciate that you're nervous, **but** you're happy to get this fixed. And that is what's important! We'll take good care of you.

Pt.   Great, thank you! It's no nice the way you guys handle your patients, **but** I'm just scared of the shot!!!

You. I get it. The shot can be scary, **but** you do have doctor gentle-hands today! You're definitely in good hands.

Pt.   Oh that's so nice to hear. I've had mostly good experiences, **but** this one time it hurt for like a week.

You. Yeah, on some rare occasions it does happen... **but** you've had mostly good experiences and today will be just one more of those.

You get the idea. We listen to what they are saying and we reframe and redirect the attention back to where we want it. We can also use "but" in the same way in our conversations, without having to reverse it on the listener. Just understanding the concept is enough to put it to work. And work, it does. Use it!

Tonality and Inflection

By now, your head might be spinning a little with a thought that goes like this: Juan, are you crazy? I didn't know I needed to pay attention to so many things at the same time in order to be a proficient communicator with my patients!

And I say: nonsense. I'm giving you MANY of the many more available concepts, ideas and techniques used to become skilled, but that doesn't mean that you need to use them all at once. It does mean if you practice with some sort of discipline, in the way I outlined at the beginning of this book, soon you'll have a wide array of tools to use when you need them.

The delivery of your s/words makes all the difference. So to piggyback on the last section, the way you use your voice is important in the effectiveness of your suggestions. The late great motivator Zig Ziglar used a sentence to explain this during his speeches. "I didn't say he stole the money."

Read the sentences below, placing the emphasis on the bold word(s), and just notice how different the meaning of the sentence is at each step.

I didn't say he stole the money

I **didn't** say he stole the money

I didn't **say** he stole the money

I didn't say **he** stole the money

I didn't say he **stole** the money

I didn't say he stole **the money**

The tonality and inflection we use when we speak has a profound impact on the meaning of the things we want to say. One of the presuppositions of NLP says that: The meaning of the communication is the response it gets

Essentially, if your listener hears something other than what you meant, YOU must adjust... not your listener. Why? Because that's the one person you have control over. You! So be aware, not only of what you are saying, but what your are conveying in the way you use your voice.

Sentence Structuring

In effective communications, **when to say what** is almost as important, as what to say. Let's use the following example to illustrate the point:

Go ahead and think about a road...

Once you have formed that image or thought of "a road", then go ahead and make it of bricks.

Lastly, to put the finishing touches on this road, go ahead and make it yellow.

Or I could have said "think of a yellow brick road". Making sure the more globally descriptive words are in front, allowing the listener to create smooth thought transitions. You see, when I ask you to think about a road I'm giving you way too much room to play... if I wanted to be vague I could talk about that road that you have great memories of. But if I want to create a specific idea in my listener's mind about a yellow brick road, I have to use descriptive adjectives and the proper order.

The issue with the road-made-of-bricks-that-are-yellow way, is not that it's hard to understand. It's that it's ineffective at leading a smooth thought pattern. It's a phrase that makes the brain start to imagine any road, and then have to come back to "correct" the image in order to make it of bricks, and then once more to make them yellow. It's jarring and it conveys lack of control on part of the speaker.

The speaker should take a moment longer to properly prepare what's about to be spoken. The extra time it takes to craft the right sentence is time saved from explanations and correcting the way things are being perceived.

As a rule of thumb, sentences should be structured from the most global descriptor to the more specific, before the subject. In the case of the example, yellow describes the bricks, and brick describes the road.

In your dental office this can play a role in something as simple as telling the patient to have a sit in your comfortable chair to something you could say during treatment, such as "find the lack of sensation from being comfortably numb... even more relaxing"

Let's take a quick look at the sample phrase and then I'll get off the soapbox about structure. In the "lack of sensation" the patient first has to wonder what will lack, and then they will experience what they believe lack of sensation feels like. An important distinction from noticing a "sensation that isn't there", where they would have to first think about a sensation and then somehow delete it, in order to comply.

And then in "comfortably numb", consider that the feeling "numb" may be pleasant for some while very unpleasant for others. So by adding a global descriptor and telling the patient HOW the numbness will feel, it allows the word "numb" (which is important) to be more easily accepted.

Intent

When I'm at a social gathering, invariably someone will ask me what I do. And when I say I'm a hypnotist, after the question of "does it work", comes the question of: How do you know how to do that?

What they would like as a response, is that there are some magic words that "make people do stuff." What they get in response from me is that the words, while important, are not as responsible for your success in hypnotic communication, as your intent to be hypnotic.

Of course I've been writing my hand off about language and the importance of the words and how they're said and when they're said and blah blah blah blah blah… Yes. But the words without the intent have a severely reduced effect, if any.

Now comes the question of how to explain intent, in a book. The answer comes to me in the form of two words: Listening, and Responding.

LISTENING: When you're intent on being hypnotic, you can adopt an attitude of 100% focused curiosity. When I say "listening" I'm not talking about just with your ears... I'm talking about being so present that your entire body and all your senses are playing a role in listening.

Being curious and allowing all your senses to be alert when communicating helps you notice things like: Body language, Breathing, Tension or Comfort in the room, which you can use for pacing and leading. Fully-present listening also gives the person you're talking to a deeper sense of connection which only helps in the hypnotic process. There's something interesting about having a conversation with someone entirely absorbed in what you're saying... have you had the experience? I encourage you to bring this attitude out with your patients. They will love you for it and you will love the results.

RESPONDING: The second portion of communicating the proper intent is to respond to what's being heard and noticed, in a way that leads the listener deeper into the experience.

Here's an example of fully-present-listening and responding when scheduling an appointment, setting up the hygienist and doctor for success with this patient:

You: Hello, welcome to _____ office, what can we do for you?

Pt: Thank you! I heard about you guys on google and then a friend also said he comes here... I need my teeth cleaned and I have tooth that's been bothering me on and off for a while. (because you asked the question and then opened up your senses to fully listen, you noticed that she used some auditory words and you also saw her make a face and shudder a little when she mentioned she needed a cleaning. So you respond and lead in the direction you desire)

You: I hear you... and thank you for coming in. I did notice the cleaning isn't your favorite part... but I can tell you _____ is so gentle, most people don't even know she's there. And the tooth that's been bothering you... tell me a little more about that one...

Pt: Sure. It hurts when I drink something cold... and some times when I chew. Ugh, I really hope she doesn't have to drill, I hate the drill! (because you were fully listening... you noticed that when she said "I hate the drill" she put her hands up to her ears as if to cover them. So you respond)

You: I understand. Well, it sounds like you may have a cavity,   some times that requires drilling but people always comment about Dr. _____'s silent drills...

Pt: What???

You: Oh yeah, Dr. _____ teaches her patients how to not hear or feel the drill. You're in good hands here. Would you like to come back after lunch today? or we have some time tomorrow morning...

In the example above you have quickly begun to calm the negative feelings surrounding this patient's visit, and you have left her wondering if Dr. X's "silent drill" will work well on her, creating expectation. That sets her up perfectly for a pleasant visit. Probably the best dental visit she's ever had, which means a loyal patient who is happy to refer friends and write reviews about you.

The best part is those referrals will come to your office already neutralized as they will have already heard about the silent drill and the gentlest hands this side of the Mississippi. It's a perfect setup that only keeps getting better as your entire team learns to work in unison with your communication skills. And here's the key to it all again: LISTEN > RESPOND. It communicates intent.

For the best way we've found to put these skills to work for you, make sure you check out our video training program: The Morning Huddle, in which we deliver the skills to your entire team and take them through a proper progression for learning these most effectively.

Free training > http://Hypnodontist.com/tmh

Applied Social Influence

Humans are interesting creatures. In many cases we act one way or another, depending on who is around or how we perceive other people's roles and the way they would deal with similar situations.

In the case of Hypnodontics, we can apply the principles of social influence to help your patients feel better, relieve pain and anxiety, let go of bad habits, and more.

Cialdini's Principles

Dr. Robert Cialdini, a professor at the University of Arizona has extensively researched and written about the 6 principles of social influence. The forces that make people act. Here is a quick explanation of each and some ways in which each is/can be used in the dental office. For a more complete understanding I suggest you read some of Dr. Cialdini's excellent work.

The 6 principles are: Social Proof, Reciprocity, Commitment and Consistency, Liking, Authority and Scarcity. In no particular order.

Social Proof: There's nothing quite as powerful as a testimonial, a referral by a patient, or seeing a busy office with happy clients. All those provide proof that you do good work, and help new patients feel confident in their decision to become YOUR new patients.

Although social proof works great in the office as one of your sales approaches, it also has practical uses in the dental chair.

You could get a patient to decide on X treatment by letting them know "most people in your situation choose X". The "most people" uses social proof and we finish it nicely with the embedded command "choose X" where X, of course, is the treatment you know is in the patient's best interest.

Any time you talk about what other patients have done and how they've acted, etc. you are applying this principle, and whether you know or not, your patients are listening for cues on how to respond. As the speaker, it is your responsibility to ensure you're positively conveying the meaning of your communication.

For example: If you go through the informed consent with your patient and you say "well some people can get dry socket after an extraction and it's very painful, but not everyone gets it", you may have just predisposed that patient to spend the next few days thinking: I wonder if I'll be one of those people that get dry socket... and where focus goes, energy flows.

A sentence that seems harmless as you read it now is not only applying social proof in the wrong direction, it's also giving the command "get dry socket" and violating the rule of speaking affirmatively with "not everyone gets it." And that's already too much working against one phrase.

You can say something that still conveys the dry socket explanation, while using cleaner and more effective language like this: "dry socket can be painful, but when people follow my instructions, they can easily avoid it. It could happen, but it's rare." - It just makes you want to be one of those people that follow instructions well, rather than one of those that gets to suffer from dry socket. Doesn't it?

Here are a few more simple phrases that apply social proof, to give you some ideas:

Talking about the needle: The doctor is so gentle, **most people** feel absolutely nothing while getting the shot.
When leading the patient: Let's take you in this room… **our patients** love this room, because the chair is so comfortable…
When distracting to give a shot: Almost every time, **patients** feel that sensation on their feet as soon as this begins to work

Stop for a moment and pay attention to the construction of the phrases above. Whatever **trigger word** we are using to apply the social proof principle becomes the open door to embed a command.

When we group the patient with "most patients, people, etc" we're giving them an idea of what is generally expected of "a person" in similar situation or under similar circumstances, and it is likely they will respond similarly.

Reciprocity: "Give and you shall receive" - enough said…

Well, not really. But that is the principle of reciprocity at its core. Doing something nice for someone can motivate them to do something nice for you.
Imagine coming back from a trip and having a friend pick you up from the airport. As you're chatting on the way home you thank him for the ride, and a moment later your friend says: Oh by the way Your Name Here , I'm leaving town this weekend and I wonder if you might be able to come over and feed my cat and make sure he's alive over the weekend…?

And then there's silence… and then most likely a definite or at least a tentative yes.

This principle can be applied in the dental office, as all these social influence principles can, by being prepared and knowing when to use them. Here are two examples:

- (For the patient that came in for an inexpensive introductory treatment) Mr. Patient, we love the patients that bring us this coupon because we find after being treated so well most want to become regular patients at our office. (I couldn't help it and used more than reciprocity there. It happens, and the compounding effect makes the communication even more meaningful.)

- (For when the doctor is about to start a new patient exam) Okay Pt. Name , we have a tradition at our office... I always promise our new patients on their first visit that I will be very gentle... as long as they choose us for all your dental needs (with a smile of course) Do we have a deal?

Commitment and Consistency: A lady approached me at a gas station a few months ago with an empty red gallon-sized tank of gas in her hand and asked if I had a quarter... I replied: No, I don't have any coins. Then she went on to say: Well actually I just need a little gas for my car and I'm asking people for quarters because it's easier. To which I replied what I think most humans would: Oh well I don't have a quarter but I can put a little gas in your tank... (and I had just loaded her weapon!) she thought that was a great idea!

As she maneuvered the tank to open it and get it ready for gas she gave me the whole back story about how she came to be in a position of having to ask strangers for money, and how difficult things were for her and her one year old being a single mother, and so on. The full on sob story. And here I am, filling up my car with $60 in gas and putting what should be 25¢ in her empty gallon tank.

What do you think I did? - Yes, I filled up her gallon of gas, basically donating over $3 to her. I knew I had stepped into her well orchestrated process when I watched her cross the street to empty the gallon in her car and come back for more. As I left the station a few minutes later her gallon was being filled by the next guy a couple of pumps over, and I imagine she made a tank of gas over the next hour or so. Not bad for an hour's work.

Before I tell you how you can use this principle in the dental office let me explain how and why this worked for her as it did: She had gently asked for help and I had made a small commitment before her sob story came out. Then, circumstances being what they were, I felt the need to remain consistent with my effort to help her and I was even aware of not wanting to feel some shame, had I stopped the fill up at $0.25 or even $1... so when she pulled on my heart strings I went all the way. It's just the way most humans are wired.

Commitment and consistency can be used effectively in confirming appointments, getting patients to adhere to instructions, presenting large treatment plans, etc. Here's an example of how I've used this principle repeatedly to effectively cut down the number of no shows at dental practices:

When calling to confirm your patients for the next day (or however long before you usually call) some times patients say they will make it to their appointment and somehow fail to show up. One thing that has helped is getting a verbal commitment that they will give you a call if their plans change. It would go something like this:

You: Hello _____, this is _____ from Dr. X's office. How are you today?

Pt: Great, thank you.

You: Excellent. _____ I'm calling to make sure you'll be able to come for your appointment tomorrow.

Pt: Oh yeah, I'll be there.

You: Perfect because we have a busy day and we want to make sure we keep everyone's schedule. Would you do me a favor... if your plans to be here change for any reason at all... can you please call me and let me know?

Pt: Of course. I wouldn't leave you hanging.

THAT is the verbal commitment. No, s/he wouldn't leave you hanging... except maybe at a time where that commitment wasn't clear.

Then this patient will want to stay consistent with their commitment so most likely they'll show up or at least call as soon as their plans change.

Liking: The social influence principle of "liking" is very simple so I won't go into much detail. It simply means you're able to influence those who like you, better than those who don't like you.

The key to taking full advantage of this principle is to become an expert at building rapport. Refer back to the section on matching and mirroring, and pacing and leading.

Authority: Dental professionals have an opportunity to use the principle of authority to your advantage every time you wear your uniform. White coats in particular have authority already built in. But any dental uniform implies authority, maybe just to a different extent, by the mere fact of showing you have specialized knowledge.

The only important thing I would like to add is that you must act the part. Your patient will give you as much respect as you're able to command. When you believe in your authority you will make them believers too. The greatest tip I can give you here is to become aware of how you use your voice. Your tone, volume, use of language, etc. have a profound effect in how much authority you project, and therefore how much you deserve.

Scarcity: Scarcity plays entirely on the law of supply and demand. Think about what happens in your mind when you're out shopping and you see a pair of shoes you like, and as you approach the rack you notice they have several pairs of the same exact shoe in all sizes and even some different colors of the same style…

By contrast, think about the same scenario except as you approach the rack you find the only pair available and lucky you it's in your size!!!

Which pair of shoes are you more drawn towards?

There are two things that let us know we're alive. One is we have a pulse… the other is we want what we can't have.

Times are changing as people become more mindful and conscious, but for most of the population it's important to make sure we get our hands on whatever is in short supply. This can be used in your practice as a limited time coupon, scheduling out a little farther in advance, or charging more for seeing Dr. X versus Dr. Z.

The beauty of it all is scarcity can have the same effect, be it real or perceived. So you must define some proper ways to inject scarcity without seeming sleazy or not genuine. The section on pre-framing will be helpful to you in this endeavor.

WANTED - Less Chemicals

One of the main reasons I decided to be an advocate for Hypnodontics was my dislike for pharmaceuticals, their side effects, and their warning labels.

I imagined a world of dentistry in which anesthetics and antibiotics were only thought of as a supplement to the resources dental patients already have inside.

Hypnosis can provide the delivery vehicle for natural anesthesia and other drugs with physiological effects. The human mind is so amazing it can produce the same effects of neurotransmitter release in the brain as the pharmaceuticals. All it needs is a compelling thought that creates the emotion that triggers it all. Which brings us to the almighty sugar pill…

Placebo

At its core, placebo uses many of the social principles outlined here. It's about "telling the lie" with enough conviction that the listener will believe in its effects, enough to make them real.

In your dental career you can be a walking placebo for all your patients, helping them feel more comfortable and influencing them to act in a way that is in line with their oral health goals. Proper communication which you're learning from this book, and our live and/or recorded training programs can facilitate a smooth operation from the moment the patient signs in at your front desk, to the moment they walk out of the door of your office happy and well cared for.

So… does the pill have to be sugar for it to be effective?

No. You can apply the effect of placebo throughout the office when everyone has the same goal in mind and is able to communicate it with the proper intent.

Remember my mentioning Dr. Gentle-hands to the patient before treatment, or asking them to pay attention to their toes to let me know when the anesthetic is working? Those are just two examples of how expectation and placebo go hand in hand.

Imagine the effect in your patients of receiving congruent communication where everything leads to a more enjoyable visit… what if none of your patients experienced pain, simply because you and your team choose to focus only on comfort and know how to properly direct the patients' thoughts to create it… what if your patients would leave quality online reviews for your practice about how caring and gentle everyone was and how their pain was eased starting with their first phone call to book their appointment? - You can achieve that and more with some practice and some synergy among your team.

Hypnodontics   Juan P. Acosta, CHP

Nocebo

At the opposite end of the spectrum of expectation we find Nocebo. As you may already be conjuring up, nocebo is created by negative suggestions that actually DECREASE the effect of chemicals and produce undesired results.

The first example that comes to mind is the patient who comes in for treatment swollen because of infection. It's obvious to you the anesthetic will have a hard time working and you know you must disclose that information… after all you want to manage the patient's expectation, right? - We're still going to do what is right by disclosing information. We're only going to change HOW the information is delivered to minimize the nocebo effect. Here's a little exercise to show you how.
Do me a favor and put yourself in your patient's shoes as you read the following statements and notice your own responses and how they differ from each other. If you were about to be treated, which statement do you feel would give you the most comfort and preparation?

First, a statement I've heard many times in similar shapes and forms:

Mr. Patient, because you're swollen most likely the anesthetic won't take or it will take a long time. So I'm going to give you a shot and we'll just wait and see, ok?

Second, a statement I'd like to hear more often:

> Mr. Patient, I'm going to give you the extra strength anesthetic since swollen tissue some times is a little more stubborn. (And then you say this as you give the patient the shot) What I need you to do is tell me when you notice the sensation on your feet, because that's when you'll know it's working already. Ok? And then we'll give it a few minutes to get really comfortably numb.

Well, what was your experience in reading these two approaches? If you're like most people, you probably experienced some resistance to the thought of going ahead with treatment on the first statement. While the second made you feel cared for, distracted you from the stubbornness of the swollen tissue, and directed your attention elsewhere for confirmation of the anesthesia via a physiological sensation that is a given. When you focus on your feet you notice them... and you notice how they feel... and because of the way it's explained it can have the effect of placebo instead of nocebo.

Here's a challenge: Stop any disbelief you may experience about the effectiveness of these simple language "tricks" and realize it may be there only because of your extensive training and the fact that going to the dentist is probably not a big deal to you, since you're in dentistry. But it is for them... you are not your patient!

So your challenge is to scan this book for those bits of language you can start to use immediately and commit to using them as often as possible.

If I were in your shoes and just learning these skills, I would select one or two things to focus on each week (or every few days) and I would start using them in a live setting. With your team, with your patients, with your friends, etc. as often as possible.

When I was getting started in hypnosis I found a job at a restaurant so I could have countless numbers of captive listeners to practice with. At first I stumbled a bit and got some funny looks… but then something started clicking and my performance sky-rocketed.

I found the compounding effect of daily practice with one or two specific skills would help me build an amazing tool box to draw from, when each situation presented itself. The result, I sold a whole lot of wine and dessert! - In fact, in only a few months I had become their lead sales trainer and consistently appeared on the top ranks when weekly and monthly performance reports came out. My average sales per person increased, the percentages of liquor vs. food, and all those things restaurants care about were coming out better than they expected, and most importantly as a sales trainer, I was able to easily spot when my coworkers and trainees were using nocebo to kill a sale and I had the tools to fix it. You don't want bad communication to kill anything... so take the challenge daily and practice practice practice.

The surest way to achieve results with the skills in this book is to create a habit of using them until they become a natural part of your conversation. Even if only to reduce nocebo, I promise you the investment of your time will be entirely worth it.

Emotional Regulation

We ask patients to calm down, yet we some times may not realize how easily our own state of mind can affect theirs.

This section is all about learning how to help someone or yourself, more easily deal with emotional ups and downs which are common in the dental office.

Managing your emotional state is a matter becoming aware of your mental state and taking some simple steps to get yourself centered.

Breathing

Let's take a moment to take a nice, really deep breath. The kind that requires a big sigh on its way out and gives you an almost instant feeling of a clearing mental state.

Breathing is one of the best tools to regulate our emotional state because since it's something we all do, we only have to learn how to use it to our advantage. Do this…

Make yourself hyperventilate by inhaling and exhaling several times in rapid succession. Do it for a few seconds.

What did you notice?

If you're human, you probably felt the increase in your heart rate and maybe even a feeling of worry or anxiety.

Now try this...

Take 10 seconds to get a full breath cycle in. Meaning one really nice and slow deep breath in and one full exhale. And do that 3 times rhythmically.

What did you experience that time?

Most humans notice a sense of calm relaxation flowing in as they breath in and a nice clearing of thoughts, kind of like a quick reboot as they exhale.

So if breathing is so important and so easily affects our emotional state, why is it not more properly taken advantage of and utilized more deliberately? The answer is lack of awareness.

Sure we have all told someone to take a deep breath and calm down, but merely saying that isn't enough to have a profound impact on the listener. What will have a deeper impact is to focus attention on the characteristics of that breath!

Meaning: instead of saying "just take a deep breath and calm down" you could use something like this:

You: Now Mr. Patient, as you take in your next, nice and deep, relaxing breath, I wonder if you're able to focus intently on the way each breath fills up your chest... and you can sort of notice it with your peripheral vision... and you might also notice how it feels as it leaves your lungs and gets exhaled with all the cares and tensions of your day...

I know it's longer. But it will save you treatment time, it will help your patient's quality of life in general, not to mention the added benefits of less impact on the treatment area, leading to faster healing times. Why? Because you and I both know a relaxed tissue will experience less damage than a tense tissue in the operatory. And less damage leads to easier healing.

Mindfulness

Many times it's easy to get carried away with a thought or feeling that ends up giving us undesirable results.

Imagine if the thoughts going through your head were: This is going to be painful; The doctor looks mean; I can't believe I have to be in traffic for an hour after this dental visit...

Thoughts such as those are bound to create negative feelings and lead to negative actions, such as canceling an appointment or simply not showing up., which hurt your practice. Ouch.

But there is something magical that happens when those unconscious thought are brought to the surface, and mindfulness exercises help facilitate this discovery.

Mindfulness can be described as my friend and colleague Dave Berman puts it: "The art of just noticing." Meaning if you were to have that thought of "This is going to be painful" you would then stop yourself as you just notice the thought and you say to yourself something like: Hmm… that's interesting… I just had a thought that this is going to be painful.

This separation from the thought, called defusion, (in mindfulness terms) as in de-fusing yourself from thoughts before they have a chance to effect emotional impact on you, provides us with an important distinction. When you have a moment of just noticing and you notice a thought as described above, you're more easily able to spot mistakes in the thinking and the way the thought is presented.

Let's analyze "I just had a thought that this is going to be painful."

When you listen to yourself noticing that thought you can challenge many things about it. And breaking it down this way allows for beliefs to change as you chip away at the thought. Sometimes it's instant. Challenging that thought would be something like this:

> Let's focus in on what "this" means... I say this will be painful, but certainly sitting here isn't... filling out the paperwork isn't... really the only thing that COULD be painful is the actual treatment, and even that sometimes isn't painful because of the anesthetic...
> I wonder why I'm thinking this is going to be painful if this is a new doctor and for all I know he's the softest, greatest doctor ever! That's silly... I should relax at least for right now. It may hurt later, but what's the point in worrying and suffering about it now?

Mindfulness exercises come in many forms. From mindful breathing to mindful eating, to imagining your mind as a railroad of three tracks and learning to catalogue your thoughts into different categories.

For the purpose of this book and keeping the flow of your practice smooth, I recommend you stick to things that are simple for you to mention in conversation as you work with your patient, instead of full on exercises.

Whatever you do, get familiar with saying: JUST NOTICE.

Anchors

Generally regarded as symbols of permanence, stability, control, etc. anchors take a new meaning in NLP terms as conditioned responses. When we create an automatic emotional response based on repetition, similar to Pavlov's dogs, we have essentially created an anchor.

There are many situations in which anchors can be used in the dental practice. For example you can help your patient re-live a moment of total comfort they have experienced before, while asking them how they feel in the dental chair.

Anchoring can be as simple as saying: On one hand (and you gesture as if you're holding something on your right) Mr. Patient, you can get the crown and feel great today... on the other hand (as you gesture with the other hand as if holding something) this temporary does give you a little time but it could start hurting. Now, if it were my mouth and I was in your situation, I would go with the crown (and gesture with the crown hand again) - What do you think you'd like to do? (and you can then gesture as if weighing their options on your hand, signaling more heavily on the crown)

When you do that, the weighing of the options, you don't have to say a word... because now they understand that your right hand is a crown and your left is waiting and possible pain.

Anchors are useful in many areas, I bet if you just think about it there are many situations in which you'd like to be able to create conditioned responses at will.

Spend a moment thinking about where in your daily life it would be useful to have a patient or team member recreate a desired emotion so they can be influenced to take the right kind of action?

Natural anchors

Anchors aren't magic, they also aren't just something we can consciously create. In-fact, conditioned responses create themselves as we go through life and experience the world around us.

Natural anchors, meaning those you haven't created at will but your patients have brought to you, can most easily be recognized by listening to the persons language and paying attention to their body movement.

A patient could come to your office and talk about the amazing weather and how amazing it is that there is no wait at your office, and all that time you, the listener, should be taking note that (apparently) "amazing" is a word that holds a strong meaning for this person. What this tells you is that later when she's in the chair you could

talk about the amazing smile she'll have in an hour and then wave goodbye to her and tell her to have an amazing day.

You see, people give us the clues we need to be able to communicate with them for maximum effect. And it is up to us to find those clues and use them to create ethical influence.

On the opposite end of anchoring maybe what your patient needs to decide on the treatment you recommend is for you to push the right buttons. Knowing what you know now, how easy would it be to help him feel a little uncomfortable, enough to get off the fence and schedule the crown, if he comes in talking about the terrible crash on the highway, or how terrible he feels about being 10 minutes late…?

That's right, it wouldn't be too difficult to figure out. You can just let him know the possibly terrible consequences of NOT adhering to your instructions or getting the treatment he needs.

Now let's take a moment to stop and take a breath. As you have gone through a good portion of this book I'm sure you've already begun to notice how this isn't about one technique or trick, and it isn't about becoming an expert, or even proficient today. What it IS about is getting your mind's gears turning so you can take the opportunity to practice these skills when appropriate.

Remember you are learning the language of ethical influence, and learning a language doesn't happen overnight.

Pain & Anxiety Relief Techniques

An important quality of the language of ethical influence is that not only can it influence decision making, but it can influence the mind/body connection to create the desired response.

In brain chemistry we learn about neurotransmitters and the way drugs like pain killers and anti-depressants affect the way they act. And as I mentioned, the same neurotransmitter release can be created without the need for chemicals.

In this section you will receive the key to your patient's mind when it comes to calming them down and helping them stop suffering from pain.

Pain is an interesting thing… it isn't one thing alone, yet so many feelings and sensations can be classified as a single word "pain." To understand how pain can be relieved it has helped hypnotherapists to think of it in terms of two distinct components, a physical one and an emotional one. In other words, there could be pain and suffering. When the suffering is relieved, the pain goes away. Below you'll find many ways to ease their suffering.

Submodalities

An image in our mind, a sound we hear, a sensation or emotion we feel, all have identifying features.

Like features on a person which make them unique, these features hold a special and unique meaning. Each meaning has been unconsciously assigned and through that association a conditioned response has been created.

For example if once you saw a spider jump and it startled you or scared you, you may have a vivid image in your mind of that spider getting closer to you, becoming bigger, and now every time you think of a spider that's the image that comes to mind…

Imagine how different the response would be if the representation you get when thinking about a spider was a little, harmless, tiny critter, walking away from you. Even if you don't have a fear of spiders, certainly you can imagine how the emotional response to the spider would be diminished in the second scenario. Can't you?

Now let's go dental… do you also think your patients might enjoy quieting the sound of the drill or being able to have the probing and scraping go unnoticed? I know they would. This is what we teach in our programs like The Morning Huddle and our live training workshops.

Submodalities come in many shapes, sizes, colors, etc. Literally, those are the types of features that make up your submodality tool box and so, they are the qualities you must ask about and pay attention to when your patients describe what they're experiencing.

Eliciting submodalities is about asking questions that get the patient to notice things they might have been unaware of up until now. You could for example have a patient interaction that goes something like this:

You.   Mr. Patient, I'm curious... when you think about the drill, is it more the noise or the way it feels...?

Pt.   Well the noise bothers me. But I just get this picture of a horror movie where the dentist is coming in really close with that tool and it's terrifying!

You.   Ah, thanks for sharing that, that helps! So when you get the visual of the dentist... does it have sound?

Pt.   Yeah! I can definitely hear the buzzing of the drill. Man it makes my ears hurt.

Ok, so far you have asked questions that told you about the buzzing sound of the drill and the visual of the dentist up close and personal with some instrument in his hand. Let's continue.

You.   Wow, it sounds terrifying. I wonder what would happen if instead you could see the dentist with a tiny instrument on his hand... way out there... (pointing at a far away spot) and I even wonder how different and much easier your experience would be if you just imagine turning down the volume of that sound... is there a volume knob or mute switch you can use?

Pt.   Hmm... I never thought about it that way, but that would be amazing!

You.   Hmm... well think about it... just for a moment... if you imagine a non-scary, professional doctor like me, with an instrument that is obviously very quiet and comfortable instead of what you used to imagine... how would that feel?

Pt.   That's interesting. It actually does feel different!

You.   Nice. Good job! Now in order to have the most amazing and comfortable appointment, what do you need to do to be able to focus only on that comfortable image?

Pt.   Hmm... I don't know.

You.   Okay, how about if we pick a spot right here... (select a spot easy for the patient to see at a moment's notice) and you can actually visualize the image of the pro (lightly pointing at yourself) with the silent instrument that's going to make your amazing smile. Would that work?

Pt.   Oh yeah. I think so. I'll give that a try!

You.   Excellent. The best thing to do is to keep that good image in your mind and whenever you need to recharge it some, you just open your eyes and see that spot. You can get those same comfy feelings right back. Fair enough?

Pt.   Absolutely. Thank you doc!

Changing the submodalities becomes a game of baby steps that compound upon each other as you build this new image/sound/feeling for your patient. Sometimes going from a loud, large drill directly to a muted tiny hand-piece is too big a jump. But you can always remember that change is change and it doesn't have to happen at 100% every time, instantly.

If you were the patient and you were rating yourself as a 7 in the discomfort scale while at the dentist, and because of some simple influential language your doctor spoke you could experience your dental appointment at a 3 on the scale... would you be mad it wasn't a zero, or would you be grateful it was better than a 7? In my experience if the patient is expecting a 7 and you can deliver a 3 you are a superhero in their mind and the 5 star reviews roll in.

Below is a list of features you can ask about and pay attention to when talking to your patients. For practical purposes of being able to work within the normal flow of your office, I recommend you stick to the two or three things that seem to hold the most meaning for your patients.

When you start eliciting and working to change lots of features it could turn into a therapy session and take too much of your chair time in production.

However, as you can see in the sample dialogue above you can combine a few of the features and weave them in and out of your conversation, navigating quickly through their thoughts and processes and helping them change. This requires _____. Lots of it. Is it worth it? In my not-so-humble opinion, every moment you invest in learning this communication style is definitely worth it.

the answer is: practice

Common features you can use

You should generally be looking for contrasting qualities you can help them adjust. Here are a few possibilities:

Colorful OR Black & White

Still image OR Movie

Close OR Far away

Loud OR Quiet

1st Person (Participant) OR 3rd. Person (Observer)

Detailed/in-focus OR Not detailed/out-of-focus

Just to name a few. Obviously they don't all need
to be used at once or used at all, for that matter

And then of course, anything else that presents itself when you ask them questions about their experience

We've found the best way to learn and internalize the language of ethical influence is to have bite sized doses to practice, without letting overwhelm take over. That's the reason we deliver our recorded training program for dental teams, The Morning Huddle in a single weekly video of about 8-12 minutes, where we give you one skill at a time and show you how to practice and implement it.

Reading these language patterns in a book is great. But being able to see and hear the way they are supposed to be used is the most valuable tool we offer. The url below will take you to our sample members page, where you can get over 45 minutes of language skills for your team before you decide whether it's a perfect fit for your team, or if they might enjoy a live training session instead.

Check out The Morning Huddle
http://Hypnodontist.com/tmh

Dissociation

Many people enjoy horror movies. Do you? Even if you don't, I'm sure you can appreciate the fact that people who like them enjoy the thrill of the movie, but most likely can only stand the fear and pain because it's on the screen. If it were happening to them in real life I would imagine they would be much less inclined to pay the $20 for pop-corn and the experience…

The language tools you are learning here and the skills you will learn from the Huddle, can help you provide your patients a dissociated experience while in the chair.

Dissociation is commonly used in the relief of pain, and fears and phobias. The simplest way I know to think about it and how to create it is to think in terms of 1st, 2nd or 3rd person.

When a person is fully associated into a memory or thought, she is in the 1st person. Seeing things through her own eyes, hearing them as she would in that moment, and feeling the emotions and sensations in her own body. She would essentially be re-living an experience, which gives the person the deepest sense of emotional connection to the memory, and therefore it's a more impactful image.

In 2nd person you may be talking to the person who is in fact going through the difficult situation (meaning pain, fear, etc) and using empathy to understand how it actually feels, as you take in the clues from their response. If they are in visible pain, the thoughts going through your head (no judgment here, just an example) could be: Wow, it looks like it sucks to be in that situation. I feel bad for them and I'm glad it isn't me.

The next step and real moments of dissociation begin when we're able to place our listener in the 3rd person. A situation which they are not part of, but just a fly-on-the-wall type observer much like watching a movie in the theater. You're watching and receiving images and sounds that create emotional responses in you, yet you know it's just a movie.

But imagine what happens then when instead of just being in the audience watching the movie, you were up in the projector room watching the audience's reactions... and how about if you were auditing the projector operator while the movie goes on... how much of the actual movie do you think you would actually catch or ever care for?

The goal with dissociation is to create space. Every step we separate the listener from "the issue" gets them closer to not caring about the issue.

In your practice you can employ dissociation with something as simple as planting simple seeds here and there as you interact with your patients. Here's a sample dialogue:

You. So what is it you're afraid of?

Pt.   Ugh, I just don't like any of it! No offense but going to the dentist just makes me uncomfortable...

You. None taken! I used to be terrified of going to the dentist... crazy huh? And now I'm here. Haha

Pt.   Wow, really? How did you get over it?

You. Well actually I watched a movie and began to notice when watching... the feelings were not as strong as they were when I thought about it being me in that chair! So when I actually had my appointment the whole time I just imagined that I was in outer-space and just watching this dentist (point to yourself) and this patient (point to them) having a nice conversation and a comfortable appointment...

Pt.   That is the craziest thing! And it worked?

You. Oh it was amazing. It worked so well that I took it one step further and imagined I wasn't even the person watching the treatment but in another space ship watching the person watching the treatment. And THAT really worked well. I know it sounds a little cuckoo but it works like a charm. Let me know how it works for you!

Pt.   That sounds interesting. And at least it gives you something to think about and distract yourself, right?

You. Yes, you can completely zone out and distract yourself! Now... where were we?

And what you have just done is created an easy process for them to follow if they choose. I believe most people, when given a choice between their original negative response and something that could work, will go for the possible gain rather than the certain failure.

Also note that by explaining the process as it worked for you in the first person, you're providing social proof and you're building rapport with the principle of liking. After all, you used to have the same fear, and look at you now!

Your goal in the thought processes you deliver should be in planting seeds and creating opportunities for the listener to discover. Most of us have a more difficult time rejecting a good idea we find on our own than one that's give to us by someone else.

Imagery

What would life be without a little color... without all the fine detail that helps us appreciate the things around us... without... well, you get the idea.

But imagery extends far beyond what we see, into the field of the imaginary and the abstract. In fact, things we feel inside our body, like the sensation of pain, can be thought of in terms of visuals.

A feeling of "pain" may seem to radiate from the center or it could feel like a blockage. Those are both useful to you when relieving pain because it's likely very easy for most of the population to add a visual representation to something radiating from the center, like a flashing red light which is brighter in the middle than the outsides. It's also likely almost if not everyone could imagine a creek which is constricted with rocks in some places or even dammed, yet free flowing in others, and it makes logical sense that removing some of those rocks would improve the regular flow of water.

So a person who is experiencing a blockage type of feeling could be relieved by using the metaphor of the creek and getting them to imagine themselves (by whatever method they find appropriate) removing those blocks or chipping away at them to increase the flow of the river. Sample language to get this started could be something like this:

NOTE: Read it all the way through first and get the feel for it. Detailed explanation follows.

You. Mr. Patient, I understand you had felt the sensation of having a sort of blockage... maybe in your circulation, that is presenting itself as "pain"... and I'm sorry. I know you want to relax and feel better of course. (pause) And it just occurred to me a buildup of pressure is similar to what happens when there's a free-flowing river, and then they build a dam in the middle of it to hold the water... and although they release some of that water on occasion and of course then the river flows free, the amount of pressure that gets built up as the water continues to grow on top of the dam continues to grow and grow... while the amount of water below the dam just flows out and there's no pressure at all... it becomes dry. Do you find you feel one side of the blockage as having more pressure than the other...?

Pt.   Hmm... yeah, I guess it feels like there's more pressure above it than below it...

You.   Hmm... I wonder what it would be like if you close your eyes and imagine opening the dam little by little, until it can begin to flow and relieve that pressure... had you thought about that yet?

Pt.   No. But I guess it makes sense...

You.   It does! You see, our mind and body are so connected you can actually create that kind of physiological change... using simple imagery, like the river, or a faucet, or even a busy highway that gets clear after rush hour. The body understands those parallels... which do you think will work best for you?

Pt.   Oh I can definitely relate to the busy highway! I love it when it clears up and you're driving and it's such a relief.

You. Yes, see!? Now I'm curious to know how much better you feel now, using that idea of the busy highway…?

Pt. Wow that's neat. I actually do feel better. Hmm…

You. Excellent! Just remember to use that anytime during the procedure and you can feel only the comfortable sensation of the free flowing highway…

But how do you know what type of imagery to use? - You ask two questions. The first one to yourself and the second one to your patient:

1) What could this compare to or what is this like? - The answer might come in the form you saw above… a flowing river, a faucet, a highway.

1) What else does it compare to or which of those works best for you? (if you've given options)

NOTE: Simply thinking about the answer begins to activate their physiology, because they can't p r o p e r l y compare and answer you without some form of test.

Then it's only a matter of feeding some enhancing details and giving them a process to follow.

Synesthesia (again)

It bears repeating and adding to synesthesia because it holds the key to many pain relief techniques.

The ability we have to "see a feeling" or "hear an image" or any other combination of senses allows us to begin to break down the sensation of pain into several tangible pieces that may on their own be less emotionally charged than the sum of all of them. In other words it helps us divide and conquer.

When you ask a patient what color they see associated with that feeling of discomfort they were experiencing, the patient has to think about the feeling from a different perspective and that is the moment when change takes place. The feeling must begin to feel differently because it now is visible. And if they were able to create that visibility I wonder how much control they have over it.

Imagine what can happen when you ask them to imagine that colored fog flowing out of their body, or the color inside where the sensation was effortlessly being painted over until it (the bad color) disappears?

Synesthesia works. Use it!

Unconscious Behaviors

It takes will power to change a belief, habit or taste. But if will power was enough nobody would visit therapists…

The language of ethical influence (hypnosis) doesn't work automatically without will power, when the time comes to change habits that don't serve us. But it does provide the boost it needs for will power to carry out and "install" the new behavior.

Changing a habit or behavior requires 3 steps I like to call the 3 Stages of Excellence. I regard excellence as the constant drive to improve and be the best we can be at that particular moment in time. So in this process we're going through we call life I say we're constantly in search of excellence. The 3 Stages: Awareness, Commitment and Action.

1) Awareness: The first step to fixing any problem is knowing it exists. Many times people realize when they are stuck in a pattern or behavior that doesn't support their goals, and many times it must be brought to their attention. Having read this far you have a great selection of tools to bring things up gently and without losing rapport, while creating change. Actually the entire book is based on that!

2) Commitment: If knowing there is a problem was the only requirement to taking care of the problem itself, the world would cease to have problems and we'd live happily ever after. Sadly that isn't the case. It takes enough emotional involvement to motivate us to follow through with the changes we desire to make.

At the commitment stage make a decision that the habit/pattern/behavior MUST change. Obviously this is the step where most fall off the wagon... but helping secure them to the wagon isn't all that difficult when you've paid enough attention to what they've communicated. If you have internalized and used the techniques in this book to elicit deeper answers from your patients, by now you know whether they want to learn to change and how they can be taught most efficiently.

If you need a review I'd recommend you check out the sections on: The direction of motivation; Applied social influence; and emotional regulation, for starters.

3) Action: The final step in the Stages of Excellence is the actual follow through. Yeah, a lot of people fall off the wagon at this station too. Why?

In my experience lack of clarity is the biggest killer of major life plans most humans have. We find it easy to say "I want to make a million bucks" or "I'm going to be president" but many times we fail to even take that goal and break it down to its most basic steps. Without doing that it's difficult to know where to start and then overwhelm takes over...

So the step of "Action" is where we break down major visions into big tasks, those tasks into simpler steps, and we can continue to dilute that vision until we reach the point where taking action is a no brainer, because by comparison the baby steps we're taking could be effortless.

A tiny sliver of change every day compounds to profound life-enhancing changes over time. The trick is finding a good balance between a step in the right direction that actually moves you closer, and one that isn't so big a step that it keeps you from taking it in the first place.

Arriving at that balance comes from a well directed question asking process. A process like funneling which you'll read about in sections ahead can help your patient negotiate through their choices, which ideally will land them in a place where they are ready to take productive action.

Once that process is in motion here's what you can do to compound its effect in the daily life of the patient.

Because unless you spend every day with your patient you must be able to give them the keys to the tools you're helping them unlock...

The compounding of a suggestion can come in many shapes. What we aim to do here is create a conditioned response that fires the right neurons during those times when they're not with us. And in order to do that I will give you three tips. Use them separately or combine them for maximum effect:

TIP #1: Attach the goodness of a new behavior, the motivating part, to an everyday occurrence for your patient. Imagine what would happen if they felt that motivation throughout the day as they see a golf course, a traffic light, or a plant at their house just because you told them they would notice the color green and how every time they noticed it they would be reminded of the great feelings that motivated them to change.

TIP #2: Make the old behavior trigger the commitment they've made. Ie: "And you'll find that any time you would have normally felt the craving/desire for X, instead of that desire you can now begin to notice the feeling that's motivating you to stick with your commitment."

TIP #3: In the tips above you have now asked them to interrupt their negative pattern and now it's time to change the direction of motivation towards their goal and keep their focus where it needs to be. On success!

Doing this is easy by planting a seed I learned to plant from my mentor and friend Scott Sandland. As a result of my training with Scott my clients now receive a patter that goes something like this: "Now and in the days and weeks to come you'll find it easy to catch yourself succeeding... and when you notice yourself take action in the right direction just like you've been aware of the issues before you can now become aware of those things which are working. And because success breeds more success, every time you catch yourself succeeding you can feel empowered and filled with wonder about what might happen the next time, and how much that success will grow with every repetition, with every day that passes and every breath you take..."

Human beings are very particular. Many times we're motivated towards a goal yet the motivation we have isn't strong enough to make us get off the couch. Either that or we didn't do a very good job at defining our action steps... but I digress. The important idea I'm going to close this section with is why "catching yourself succeeding" is so important. Humans won't always go for what they desire, but they will always defend what they already have.

Meaning if they feel they have begun to make changes they will expect the changes to continue. And expectation is the precursor of lasting change.

The Con Artist

The Con Artist's job is to make believe in such a convincing way that the person being conned is none the wiser.

Because people are skeptical when it comes to believing what they think and say, this has a profound effect in the results they achieve. I find it important to be very aware of the concept of pre-framing you learned much earlier in this book, and take your listener through a scenic route of their liking.

When I started learning hypnosis my first interest was performing comedy skits in front of large audiences. Using a combination of hypnosis, magic and "mind reading" skills, audiences were taken from their current reality into a new realm of possibility and awe for the immense potential of the human mind. After the shows I would have people from the audience come up and ask if I could help them quit smoking or lose a few pounds. So the show was a scenic route to getting the hypnotherapy work.

Had I put an ad out for stop smoking hypnosis I might end up with zero business from it... Except I did do that and I did get zero. But because at the show they were exposed in the way THEY wanted to be exposed now the door was open for me to offer them more.

Being in a position of "control" and authority brings out an element of compliance and puts you in the driver's seat for this experience you're going to give your patients. Your patients have volunteered to come to your show. They are paying to see you and get the results they desire.

As the expert and their guide, it is your job to properly communicate the illusion of choice so your patients are funneled where you want them.

For a complete training solution for your entire team for pennies a day check out The Morning Huddle

The Hypnodontist™ complete video training program complete with worksheets, homework and easy anywhere access, delivered to you in easy-to-watch 8-12 minute training segments

http://Hypnodontist.com/tmh

Apendix: Dental Phone Script Book

Hypnodontist.com

Dental Practice Optimizer

Dental phone skills 911
(version 001.2)

Introduction

In this report we will talk about the best phone practices for the dental office.

Over the last few months I've had the privilege of working with many dental practices and arriving at similar situations at most of them. They know they're leaving lots of money on the table because they don't have a proper selling system in place, and worse, they don't know how to make it better. Their stories generally come from the doctor's mouth like this:

We have a long list of patients that we've offered treatment to, who haven't booked yet… We have new patients coming in for an inexpensive exam or cleaning and can't seem to turn them into patients for the Tx we offer… We have 2 or 3 open spots in hygiene almost daily and we have tons of patients we could be scheduling… etc.

In most of these cases I have tracked down the issue to less-than-great communication skills. One thing that is important to understand is that this isn't about anyone doing something wrong, because in my experience most front desk and office staff members are competent and possess excellent people skills. This is ONLY about OPTIMIZING your results. Meaning making better something that is already good.

This is a growing body of work which I will continue to develop for you to create a comprehensive set of tools to help you grow your practice exponentially. Parts of this script book may also be found in my book "Hypnodontics: Ethical Influence Language for Dental Professionals", being released in Summer 2014.

Okay... we have appointments to book, practices to grow and team members to congratulate on their exceptional performance. So we better get started.

Speaking your patients' language

One place where professionals in most fields can improve, is understanding that official and slang dentistry terms aren't for their patients. They're for their staff and other dental friends.

Telling your patient she needs a "Prophy" isn't a good way to start your conversation. If you get to the point of calling it that after explaining it that's okay, but for the greeting portion and initial offer you will get more value out of calling it a cleaning and explaining the benefits of it, than "saving time" and calling it by its nickname: Prophy.

Prophy is just an example. I simply want to encourage you to speak in easy to understand terms and to normalize the patients' experience as much as possible. Remember they didn't do to dental school and what to you is a simple routine procedure might be a nightmare for them, and much worse if they don't understand it.

Funneling your patients

Think about a world in which the patient tells you what they can or can't/want or don't want to do...

Nice, I know!

Well that's what "funneling" is all about. Creating the right opportunity for the patient to self-select and either buy in, or let you know they won't.

In funneling I will teach you how to best present the options to the patient. This section is broad because EVERY INTERACTION that you have with a patient should direct them where you want them to go. Here are some examples:

You get a call from a patient who wants to change his cleaning appointment... you now have to deal with an open spot in tomorrow's schedule, and push the patient to come in and you're on a really tight schedule. (if you're not on a really tight schedule, you need to make it seem as if you are. Chair time is a dental practice's life-line.)

So instead of throwing out responses like: Okay, I have a spot on Tuesday at 5 or Wednesday 10am but you might have to wait a little while on Wednesday because we're pretty booked.

You can start by handling the objection of having to wait like this:

DT (Dental Team Member): Okay, I have a few spots open in the next couple of days, some are a little tighter on the schedule… would you prefer to maybe have to wait a little, or to have one of the other spots where we can almost guarantee no wait?

Weird? Here's why. This takes the stress out of your schedule when he says: I don't mind waiting, or I don't want to wait. Since you've already told him there are those two options, you have now limited the options in the scheduling and created scarcity. If the patient says he doesn't mind waiting, you can fill in a spot that needs to be filled. And if he says he needs a more set appointment, then the choices you offer will have to be more appealing now that they know the other options are "waiting" options. It's simple supply and demand… we limit availability slightly to properly motivate them and get them to where we want them to go.

Understanding these skills isn't about a one time victory. It's about an attitude of staying a few steps ahead of the listener so you can pull the right strings of motivation for them.

Throughout the rest of this script book keep in mind that EVERYTHING YOU'LL READ here fits under the umbrella of funneling and efficiency at the office. Doing the things that are most valuable and would mean most to the success of the practice, at every step of the way.

Getting them to upgrade from their first visit's introductory offer to paying client

You put time, effort and money into getting a postcard, ad, commercial, etc. into the eyes and hands of potential dental patients. All of a sudden you receive a nice influx of patients, coming for very inexpensive or even free services, and you're faced with the "follow-up" call to schedule them for treatment.

You know, because you're smart, that most patients that come in aren't going to convert into a $7,000 treatment plan, but you are willing to play the numbers game. Here's how to improve your odds DRAMATICALLY.

By the way, this is something you can do in person during the original treatment plan presentation (before they blow you off to "think about it") but for the purpose of this book of "phone" scripts, I'll stick to the format.

Follow this exercise: Put yourself in the patient's shoes… you've come in for the incredible value of a free (or inexpensive) exam/cleaning… you know there's probably something wrong with your mouth but you can't seem to make it to the dentist (for whatever reason), and today you will because it's free and you have to take advantage of that! Fair enough. During your exam the doctor rattled off a few things to his assistant, and when they were done they showed you a huge list of things they'd like to do to your mouth for only $7,000.

That's an exercise in pacing. Pacing is being able to meet your patients where they are mentally and emotionally, before you lead them in the direction you want them to go.

Pacing and leading as a technique for effective communications, is valuable in every area on your practice. I don't use generalizations lightly… and I have to tell you that EVERY interaction with a patient must be wrapped around the concept of pacing and leading, in order to be a successful, win/win situation.

When I approach dental offices to offer Hypnodontist™ DPO services I hear doctors and other DTs tell me they hate sales and don't want to be high pressure. And the reason most people don't like "sales" is because they don't like to be pushed and understandably, they don't want to be the ones causing that uncomfortable feeling in others.

There's nothing wrong with not wanting to be high pressure. There is something wrong with knowing your job depends on sales, and not looking for a way to learn how to sell predictably AND without pressure.

In most cases, that follow-up call to offer treatment after an inexpensive or free service sounds something like this: (IF they pick up…)

Dental Team Member (DT): Hi {pt. name}, this is {your name} from {your office name}. How are you today?

Patient (PT): Great thanks.

DT: Oh good! (with a really high pitched voice) I'm just calling to follow up after your visit and to see if we can schedule you in for treatment...

PT: Umm... (click)

Or...

PT: Oh yeah, I can't pay for all that... and I don't have insurance...

Or...

PT: {Anything else they can say to blow you off}

And in some cases...

PT: Oh yeah, I haven't had a chance to call you... can I come in maybe Tuesday of next week?

Sound familiar?

So the patient is enjoying her day, completely unaware of your existence, and all of a sudden she's put in the uncomfortable position of having to be vulnerable. She has to open up to you and explain about her finances, or she has to tell you she had no intention to ever move forward with treatment but still told you she might. As soon as they realize where the call is from the defenses go up, unless they are in-fact ready to be treated.

I hope from the patient's perspective you can see how the sample call above could feel like an attack! It's too direct, it's too fast, it doesn't follow the proper process of disarming and building rapport before asking for money. Really, that's what that call is for... to ask for money. And even if your heart is in the right place, which I've found in most cases it is, it sounds detached and impersonal, and it makes it easy for people to say no and feel justified.

In the following phone greeting and funneling sample, pay attention to how gently we move the patient through the process and let them tell us how to proceed. This is proper hypnotic sales technique, and it's about as low pressure as sales can be. Read it first as if you were the patient.

DT: Hi {Pt. name} this is {your name} calling from {your office name}, how are you today?

PT: Great, thanks.

DT: Good. {Pt. name}, you came to our office last {day/date/etc} and we showed you a big treatment plan... we know that most times people come in for an exam and don't expect that, so I'm calling to see if I can help you prioritize that list. Do you have any questions, or was there a specific part of the treatment you thought you'd start with?

PT: Yeah, it was so much stuff I'm kind of lost...

DT: I understand... that's why we call! So let me ask you... tooth #15 towards the back right and 31 on the other side both need work. Is one of them bothering you more than the other or about the same?

PT: No, actually neither one of them is hurting... yet.

DT: Ah! Lucky! Haha... so then it comes down to preference. It looks like 15 is going to be a little more involved since it's a {treatment}... We recommend you start with that one because of that, but ultimately it's up to you. Do you have a day next week that would work best?

PT: Umm... yeah, that sounds good. I would prefer Tuesday if you have anything open.

DT: Ok, let me check... umm... Tuesday... I have... the schedule is a little tight, I have a 10 and a 3, but the morning is busier so you may have to wait a little. Would you prefer that or the 3pm with almost or no wait?

PT: Yeah, I don't mind waiting. Let's go with the 10am.

DT: Great, {Pt. name}. I'll give you a courtesy call Monday to remind you of your appointment and we look forward to your visit on Tuesday.

Let's debrief that call and then I will give you an assortment of responses below, because I realize that the above patient isn't a particularly difficult patient. Remember all I'm asking you to do is listen more closely to what they want and guide them through the options in a logical and understandable way.

Notice how most of the DS responses above do something to agree with or pace the patient, and then take her to the next step by ending with a question. Ending with a question gives you control over the conversation.

The greeting is disarming because it doesn't call to schedule her for treatment, but to help her prioritize her choices and answer any questions.

The script gently gives the Pt. the illusion of choice throughout, where any choice is still a good choice for the patient and for the practice. This work is all about creating win/win situations. After all, you entered the dental field because you too want what's best for the patient.

Using humor in your calls in a way that's natural for you is highly recommended. With proper timing and delivery, humor can be the fastest way to build rapport and compliance. When humor is used in conjunction with the right motivator, like in the example above when DS says "Lucky!" about the patient having no pain yet, it can strengthen your connection and open the door for the next suggestion.

Pay close attention to how the script above keeps the forward motion by dealing with one thing at a time (pacing) and then asking a question that moves them to the next thing without missing a beat (leading).

LEADING => FUNNELING meaning when you lead the patient you are asking them to self-select and tell you what works for them so that you can simply provide it. It's the ultimate in customer service and the softest way to sell.

Here are some sample responses:

PT: No, I don't have any questions, thanks.

PT: Umm… yeah I don't think I'll be scheduling…

PT: Haha! You guys showed me $10,000 worth of treatment after a free exam and you want me to just come in and get it done?

PT: Well my {tooth} is hurting so let's start with that one.

PT: Actually no. I just came in because the exam was free/cheap but I have no intention of scheduling.

PT: I'd love to come in but I don't have the money right now.

PT: {anything else that you hear as an initial objection regarding money, schedule, service, insurance, etc.}

In the resource section at the end of this script book you'll find an organized list of possible responses back, since Pt. responses and objections will be similar in many of the conversations you'll have.

NO Message

I suggest there are only 2 messages that you should leave in a Pt's voicemail on the first call: The appointment confirmation or courtesy call message, and a message to a "dead list" meaning patients that haven't been here for a long time so we don't know if they're still patients at our practice or have gone somewhere else.

For follow-up, to sell treatment, or to discuss anything else that may have to include a new discussion about money, insurance, anxiety, etc. I recommend calling until they answer (over a period of time of course) or until it just becomes clear they're blowing you off (3 calls) before leaving a message. Below you'll find the messages you can use in these cases. The focus of these calls is to sell treatment and fill up Hygiene so your practice can move faster from surviving to thriving.

Appointment confirmation messages

Confirming that patients will come in for their scheduled time is one of the key elements of a successful dental practice. A patient that doesn't stick to his appointment takes a VERY LARGE portion of the day's income to the practice.

At first, when you have scheduled a free or inexpensive appointment one might think: well, it's not that big a deal, it's not like they were going to be paying a lot and probably not even doing treatment afterwards. Good riddance…

And that is dental practice death for several reasons:

- There is no new patient to possibly enroll in continuity programs or offer treatment to.

- The high demand doctor's time is now being wasted. As well as anyone else.

- There isn't even that little bit of income coming from them… every little bit helps.

- There's huge opportunity loss. Meaning another paying Pt. could have been in the chair then.

- And of course it just rolls downhill because a struggling practice can't pay the same or care the same.

So the key thing to understand here is that we must maximize chair time at all possible times. And the best way to do that is to ensure that the patient that's supposed to be in it shows up!

Let's take a look at two of the principles of influence that can motivate a patient to call back about their appointment, and keep the time you originally gave them.

Scarcity: The lack of something, or even better… the perceived lack of something.

Reciprocity: The mutual back-scratch. I do something for you and you can do something for me.

So a sample message goes like this:

DT: Hi {Pt. name} this is {your name} calling from {your office name}. The reason I'm calling is because we have a really tight schedule {tomorrow/on Thursday/etc} and I'm calling to make sure all our patients will be on time.

We have you scheduled for a {free cleaning/introductory exam/x-ray and check-up} for {exact time}. If your schedule has changed or you can't make it for any reason… Would you give me the courtesy of a call back so we can update our calendar?

Thanks so much and we look forward to seeing you tomorrow! Talk to you soon. {hang up}

That message creates the impression that you have no time to spare (and hopefully that's true, but even if it isn't yet, this will help make it so.) It gets them thinking about calling you and about being on time, not just about being there, which further shows you're a busy office.

Then the message asks for a courtesy call back. You are giving them the courtesy of a confirmation call and expect them to return the nicety. It also shows them you are serious about them keeping your schedule if you're making sure all your patients will be on time, and it does all those things directly and gently.

There's nothing for the patient to complain about. And if they are planning to not show, the extra bits of motivation can make them pick up the phone to let you know.

I'm sure you can agree the difference is night and day with the following, sort of standard message left by most:

DT: Hi {Pt. name} this is {your name} form {your office name}, just calling to confirm your appointment for {day} at {time}. Please give us a call if you have any questions, otherwise we'll see you {day}

I know it's hard to compare apples and oranges... but if you could... this would be a similar comparison. The first message gets results and call backs. The second gets missed appointments and your office's money flies out of the window via an empty dental chair.

When the patient picks up the phone you can use virtually the same greeting as if you were leaving a message, with the one big difference that you must be on your toes and ready to respond in real-time.

Dead list message

A dead list isn't where you want to spend lots of time on a recurring basis. So it's best to guide these patients to quickly sort themselves out as either potential patients, or not interested.

So the message below is designed to relieve the interpersonal tension that might build from having to say "no" to you, build rapport, and it also give them a sense of urgency, so that if they are considering coming back they will do it soon.

DT: Hi {Pt. name} this is {your name} from Dr. {last name}'s office. We haven't seen you in a long time and I'm giving you a quick courtesy call to see if… maybe you started working with another dentist, or if it's time to schedule you for an evaluation or cleaning…

When you call me back please have a date in mind for your appointment. We have a few spots open over the next couple of weeks so we should be able to see you fairly soon.

Thanks for your time and I would really appreciate a quick update so we can take care of you properly, or update our records if you've gone elsewhere.

I look forward to your call. Have a great day. Bye now.

As you can see, the message is disarming and stops wasting everyone's time. If the patient was not only a routine patient but has lots of treatment presented, I suggest not leaving a message initially because it makes it too easy for them to avoid you.

In that case, I'd recommend a few calls and hang-ups before leaving a message. And then that message could go like this:

DT: Hi {Pt. name} this is {your name} from Dr. {last name}'s office. We haven't seen you in a long time... and I'm calling to see if we can get a quick update from you. I'm guessing maybe you're working with another dentist, or maybe now you're ready to get started with some of your treatment. I know we gave you a long list so... The least we can do is help you prioritize it.

Thanks for your time and I would really appreciate a quick update so we can take care of you properly, or update our records if you've gone elsewhere.

I look forward to your call. Have a great day. Bye now.

Or something along those lines…

I hope you're getting the understanding that there is no right or wrong with these calls, as long as you follow the basic steps of pacing, and leading. If you put yourself in the shoes of your patient receiving such a call, what do you think would be going through your mind, and what is it that you would need to hear to motivate you to return the phone call one way or another? - That's the perspective you should adopt when getting on the phone.

The 3 Ps.

Proper Patient Preparation

This is one of the crucial pieces of phone work that can boost the success of your practice tremendously. Proper patient preparation on the initial phone call brings many benefits to the practice and to the patient. Here are some of those:

- Patients may require less chemical anesthesia.

- Patients may experience less pain and discomfort.

- Patients will suffer less anxiety and stress prior to their scheduled appointment.

- Patients can feel well cared for and it ratifies the trust they've put in you and your practice

- Your practice will enjoy higher ratings and better/ more reviews and word of mouth referrals.

- Your practice will experience less resistance during the sales process.

- Your practice will dramatically reduce the number of no shows.

- Your practice will increase retention and loyalty, creating long term relationships with your patients.

The even better news is: preparing patients for their appointment is so easy! All you have to do is make sure you cover a few bases as if following a recipe:

(The order in which you put these isn't vitally important. But you must ensure there's a natural flow, and as you funnel the patient you should have gathered all the info you need to craft your closing statement for every time a patient calls to schedule)

- Confirm day of the week, date and time.

- Inject a little scarcity. In other words, put a little light under them to make sure they make their scheduled time.

- Use reciprocity for a little leverage.

- Get a VERBAL commitment.

Here's an example that follows that recipe:

DT: Ok {Pt. name} we're going to take really good care of you, I have your appointment set for next {Day} the {Date} at {Time}. I will call you to confirm anyway, but as of right now would there be any reason why you might not make it to your appointment?

PT: Nope, that sounds good. Thank you!

DT: Great! We look forward to seeing you then. We're booked pretty solid that day, so if you're able to make it a few minutes early that would ensure there's plenty of time for you to sign in and be ready for your {Time} spot. If for any reason you think you may be running late or not able to make it, will you give us the courtesy of a phone call? (AND SHUT UP AND WAIT FOR THEIR COMMITMENT)

PT: Absolutely! I wouldn't leave you hanging.

DT: Excellent. That's all we ask! You're all set then, see you {Day}. Enjoy the rest of your day.

And here's another:

DT: Alright {Pt. name}, you're all set to see Dr X {Day, Date, Time}. Our schedule is pretty tight that day so I will be calling you the day before to make sure we all stay on schedule so you don't have to wait long. If anything changes with your schedule in the meantime it isn't a big deal... as long as you can give me a call and let me know at least 24 hours in advance. Can I count on you to do that?

PT: Oh yeah, for sure. (and so on…) you get the idea, right?

If they're not very sure they can call you back that's a clear sign that they may just skip your appointment. You MUST probe for answers until the patients themselves are certain they are coming.

Mishaps happen and schedules sometimes get messed up. That's normal. But if you get a verbal commitment the likelihood of them at least calling you back if they need to change their appointment goes up exponentially.

The next portion isn't necessarily a phone technique, but it can be. I'm going to give you a few nuggets of info you can use to prepare your patients when they arrive at your practice, and if you wish to do so over the phone, it works just as well.

Here are a few things you can use to achieve the desired results described in the benefits above. Some have sample things to say:

- Use the quality of the dentist and the dental work to get the patient excited.

DT: You are in excellent hands. Dr. X is so nice and so gentle… so don't be too surprised if your appointment is enjoyable!

DT: You're so lucky to have Dr. X. We will take really good care of you {Pt. name}, we look forward to seeing you on…

- Use humor to relax the patient.

DT: You can be confident you'll have a great appointment. Patients say Dr. X has the gentlest hands this side of the Mississippi… haha.

DT: Now you can just relax as I put this fashionable x-ray vest on you!

DT: Whatever other corny line you want to throw in that can help break the tension patients may be feeling about their appointment.

- Use statements to normalize things and desensitize the patient. (you can pepper these in during your conversation, where they fit comfortably)

DT: It is an easy routine procedure.

DT: We do so many of those. (referring to X treatment)

DT: Our patients say that all the time, and then they come for their appointment and are amazed at how great it was!

- Build rapport by remembering small details. (take notes on things that might be important to the Pt. Family, pets, friends,

- Forecast what's going to happen. (lightly)

DT: So when you come in {day of the week} the Dr. will spend a few minutes making sure your nice and comfortable, and then he'll do what he does best.

- Work on getting good reviews starting with the first phone call. If the opportunity arises to mention your great online reviews, do so.

- Find out what's important to that patient and remember to do your best to provide it.

- Be empathetic. Put yourself in the patients' shoes.

- Listen, listen, and then listen some more.

- Use stories. Stories sell... Do you remember another patient with the same issues, the same Tx, etc? Make sure it's a success story.

Be flexible with your approach. Some patients require lots of phone time, some very little. What's important here is that you get a feel for the patient and what they are communicating without saying it... do they sound wishy washy on the phone about keeping their appointment? They probably are.

Half-alive list outbound calls

Calling patients that came in for something inexpensive or free a long time ago and were offered treatment, but

haven't scheduled. Meaning these are "non-performing" patients. A "dead list."

When calling a dead list, the most important objective of the call is to determine if the person is an actual potential patient of the practice. It's much more cost effective to receive a quick "no" and let the patient off the hook, than to spend valuable phone time trying to reach them every month to follow-up, only to be blown off by them... they're not interested. Let them go.

So here's how a greeting to these patients could go:

DT: Hi {patient name}, this is {your name} from {your practice's name}. How are you this morning/afternoon/etc?

PT: Oh hi... I'm good. Thanks.

DT: The reason for my call is after your visit to our office in {month/year/whatever} we showed you a long-term treatment plan (only say long-term if it's a BIG treatment plan) and I'm calling to see if we can help you start with the things that are most urgent like {the 2 fillings, the crown, the X...} or if you've already had work done elsewhere...?

(AND THEN YOU STAY QUIET AND WAIT FOR A RESPONSE.)

(This greeting technique effectively gets them off the hook if they don't want to be your patient, or gets them thinking in the direction of getting scheduled for at least a portion of the treatment offered. If the treatment plan isn't extensive enough to break it up in small pieces for them, you can use recurring services as the second choice. Meaning a cleaning, Bwx and exam, or... anything. The idea here is to give the illusion of choice, when in reality any answer is a benefit to you.)

Here are some sample possible responses:

PT: I did get started working with someone else…

PT: Oh no, I do want to come in but I have this problem with my insurance…

PT: Haha! You guys showed me $10,000 worth of treatment after a free exam and you want me to just come in and get it done?

PT: Yeah, that would be great! I got so lost not knowing where to start with so much to do in my mouth…

PT: Actually no. I'm not able to pay that so I don't think I'm coming.

PT: Oh no, I'm so freaked out of going to the dentist, and last time I was at your office it hurt!!!

PT: {anything else that you hear as an initial objection regarding money, schedule, customer satisfaction, insurance, etc.}

Does that phone call seem counter-intuitive to you?

That phone call is designed to uncover their objection quickly so we can deal with it. Additionally, if they don't want to come in but would be embarrassed to say so directly, we are giving them an easy out so we can stop wasting their time AND ours in calling them incessantly to try to schedule.

Think about this and for the duration of this book of scripts PUT YOURSELF IN THE PATIENT'S SHOES on the other end of the line. You came in for a free exam or a 100 dollar cleaning a year and a half ago, at which time the doctor told you your mouth needed $4000 worth of treatment and tried to get you to make a decision about getting it done. You told them you would look at your schedule and think about it, because you don't want to feel embarrassed to say that you're just not ready to pay 4k for optimal dental health at this time (for whatever reasons).

Then you get a phone call out of the blue from a dentist's office you may or may not remember, and what they give you as a greeting is: Hi this is ___ from ___ office and I'm calling to follow up on your visit to our office a year and a half ago. Wondering when we can schedule you for treatment...?

Let that sink in...

That is B A D bad. It puts the patient in the sad position of having to lie to save face, and the dental practice suffers the hit of using valuable employee hours on someone who is not interested.

What happens if it hasn't been that long since they came in? Maybe it's been only 30 days and they haven't scheduled their appointment. People in this group can be transitioning to the "blowing you off" group, but they could also be in the "I haven't had enough time to digest this, get my ducks in a row, and call you" category. Meaning these are probably more likely to buy, and also have you in mind a little more because of recency.

The technique is similar, with the exception that you may be able to be more direct about asking to schedule an appointment since it is probably expected by the patient to receive a follow-up call. The greeting and call can go like this, played out here, objections and all:

DT: ... I'm calling to answer any questions you might have and schedule your next appointment. Do you have any questions?

PT: No, I'm just not ready to schedule yet...

DT: Okay, not a problem. Do you have a time-frame in which you'd like to get started with your treatment, so that I'm not bothering you by calling too often?

PT: We'll actually I'm just not sure I'm going to schedule at all… I just got my insurance and it doesn't take effect for another 60 days.

DT: I understand, that happens a lot. Well let me ask you… if there was a way to get treated before your insurance kicks in, would you rather wait or take care of it now?

PT: Oh yeah, if it wasn't for the insurance thing I'd be in there for sure!

DT: Oh okay. Something that works well for most patients in this situation is using a {your payment plan} account which has no interest or payments for {X number} of {days/months}, as a bridge so they can get treated right away, and by the time their payments are due they have a head start on the insurance. Would you like me to check if {your payment plan} is an option for you?

PT: No, my credit is terrible…

DT: I hear that all the time, that's not a problem… We've found that these companies seem to finance a lot of people that don't think they can get financed. Let me ask you… do you have a steady income or someone that might be able to help you as a cosigner?

PT: Yeah, I have a job… it's just my credit…

DT: Well, if you have a job it's worth going through the application. Can't hurt…

PT: Yeah but if I don't get approved my credit will be even worse from checking it.

DT: Ok, I understand. It sounds as if the fear of losing a point of credit is worse than the toothache! Haha… not a problem. Please give us a call back when you decide we can help you.

Etc… etc… etc…

Yeah, I took you all the way down the rabbit hole in that one… it happens. Learn to lead the patient down that hole as quickly as possible by not letting them give you half answers that don't commit them to anything.

If they are going to say "no", we want them to actually say "no" so we can be done and move to the next patient. It isn't about forcing treatment and routines on everyone, it's about finding those who are ready for treatment or routine appointments.

Get a commitment

A major killer of productivity when making phone calls to patients is allowing them to get off the hook too easily. And it's an issue of DT feeling uncomfortable about asking direct questions. Fair enough.

Asking direct questions of another person can be a little unnerving until you understand how it is the most beneficial approach for all parties involved. A direct question doesn't have to be mean or come out rough. It needs to be presented with the curiosity of fact finding and the intent of saving everyone time down the road.

Why? Because your time is valuable. Doing this and getting even the small commitments throughout the process is the best policy to ensure efficient use of your resources.

There's something that happens inside a person when a commitment is vocalized. Think about this conversation as if you were the patient:

PT: Yeah, I'm not sure I'm ready to schedule... I'll call you back.

DT: Ok, not a problem. Do you know when I can expect your call? (and then stay silent and expect a response)

PT: Umm... I will call you by Tuesday/the end of the week/next month...

DT: Ok excellent {Pt. name}, I look forward to your call. Have a great day.

But what if they respond differently...

PT: Haha... what, you need me to tell you when exactly I'm going to call you?

DT: Haha not exactly… what I mean is I don't want to be wondering if I should call you back if it's too soon. So I just want an idea of your time-frame…

PT: Oh I see… haha. No problem. I think I'll get it done in the next couple of weeks.

DT: Perfect. Thank you for your time {Pt. name}, and I look forward to your call. Have a great day.

There's always a way to put a positive spin on whatever you ask of a patient. All actions must have a perceived benefit to the patient. And also notice on the mismatched response above where the PT laughs at our question, that DT starts by pacing the laugh and relieving the tension of the mismatch by creating the illusion of a "misunderstanding" and moving on to explain a benefit to the patient even if it's minimal.

A broken fifty thousand dollar machine

One day while working at the clinic and handling the appointments we had a panoramic x-ray machine stop working. All of a sudden we were not only losing a fair amount of money on every single patient we couldn't x-ray, but we also had to use the PA machine which was less comfortable for the patient and it put the staff in the also uncomfortable position of having to explain why our expensive piece of equipment wasn't working. Not the best feeling for the patient who was trusting us with their care, if you think about it from their perspective.

It was a busy weekend and there was no way to get the machine fixed until next week, so I prepared myself to make lemonade from the lemons we had available and started looking for ways to say things to the patient on the phone that would turn the mishap of the broken machine into a benefit to them.

It took me a few phone calls to get the concept right, and I'm sure you'll find that as you put these skills to the test you'll be fumbling at first and then becoming smoother and more natural. But when it clicked it was probably my best piece of phone work to date.

After taking the patient through the entire explanation of our services (as if the machine was working, prices and all) the calls went something like this:

DT: Hey {Pt. name} let me ask you... did you say it's a {bottom left molar/front tooth/wisdom tooth/etc.}? Because we may be able to save you some money IF the doctor can take just the handheld x-ray...

PT: Yeah, it's a {bottom left molar/front tooth/wisdom tooth/etc.} and that would be great!

(Keep in mind that this was an emergency dental clinic with a limited range of services and out of insurance network, so using money as the motivation is strong. In reality, money is a big deal at most practices and one of the main objections for actually booking appointments I hear. But what's important for you to understand is how I used the scenic route to their deeper motivation to help the doctor and the practice save face. Not only that but we received reviews because there isn't a happier customer than a customer that truly believes he/she received a tremendous value. Any time a "sales person" downsells a prospect it breaks a pattern and creates a whole new set of emotions for the prospect)

DT: Yeah it would! Well listen… all you have to do is ask Doctor X when you're there if he/she might be able to do the handheld x-ray. That way you'll only pay X instead of Y!

PT: That's amazing! Thank you so much!!!

When I initially devised this call the doctors were not aware… and it was really fun to hear some of them talk about the interesting phenomenon happening that weekend where patients (almost as if they knew) were coming in asking for the PA x-ray.

The money we had lost because of the broken machine was gone anyway. The only way to mitigate further damage to the clinic was to create the right emotion in the patient, and that was the emotion of excitement at the prospect of saving some money on their x-rays. This allowed the doctors and staff to not have to shamefully admit our equipment was broken and it also led to increased patient satisfaction and word of mouth in the form of online reviews.

Luckily, instead of only mitigating the damage, this particular approach turned our issue into an advantage of the patient. And that pays off any day of the week.

Possible responses by them
and counter-responses by you

Writing scripts is a funny thing because everyone can read a script in different ways… so the samples below fit my style and the way I ACT in my patient interactions. Meaning the pauses I use, the body language, etc. Please read them and understand their INTENT. And then spend a few minutes making them your own. A little upfront preparation will turn your results from haphazard treatment sales, into a predictable sales process, that as an added bonus increases patient satisfaction and retention. Why? Because they're not being pushed and sold directly but through the whole process we're giving them the illusion of choice. Where every choice is a good choice.

That being said, in the next few pages you'll find the possible responses that I've given through the examples in this report, with a sample counter-replies by DS that either funnel the patient properly, sell treatment, get them off the hook, or {your benefit here…}

*These are in no particular order. Please read them and craft some of your own!

PT: I did get started working with someone else…

DS: Ok, that's fine. We wanted to make sure you were taken care of. If you ever need us please call…

(Nothing you can do here and stay within professional ethics, except to be very polite and express to them you'd like to be their office of choice if they need you.)

PT: Actually no. I'm not able to pay that so I don't think I'm coming.

DS: I understand. We do offer a payment plan option and take most insurance plans… Is there something we can do to help take good care of you?

(This gives them the opportunity to blow you off clean if that's what they wanted to do in the first place, and gives them options if they're sincere)

PT: I'd love to come in but I don't have the money right now.

DS: I understand. Let me ask you though… if money wasn't an issue would you get your teeth taken care of? Because we do have some really good payment plans, we can help with your insurance… etc.

(this helps you decide if they will ever be a patient of if the money objection is just their way of blowing you off)

PT: Oh no, I do want to come in but I have this problem with my insurance…

DS: I know… we deal with so much insurance. Would you like me to help you figure it out so you can come in or is there anything else stopping you from getting the treatment you need?

(This is designed to just be helpful and to flush out the objection if it wasn't their only reason for rejecting you.)

PT: No, I don't have any questions, thanks.

DS: Ok great! Do you have your schedule handy so we can find a time that works for you, or would you like me to call you back {later today/tomorrow/at 3pm next Friday…}

(The idea is to push them as far as they need to go to actually be truthful and tell you they're blowing you off, or to book the appointment. This particular response and any other dry or "dead" response is best dealt with directly, understanding that this particular patient isn't yours to begin with. Meaning there's nothing to lose. Stop wasting your time and theirs.)

PT: Oh no, I'm so freaked out about going to the dentist, and last time I was at your office it hurt!!!

DS: Oh I'm sorry to hear about that. And they usually call me/him/her Dr. Gentle Hands... haha. The good news is that now we're working with a Hypnodontist and he helps a lot with the fear, anxiety, etc. Would you like me to see when he'll be here next so we can schedule you?

(Being empathetic and helpful goes a long way in the dental office. Many times we think that because we see root canals and extractions every day they're normal routine for everyone and what we say some times may sound as if we're discounting their concern. So the formula here: Pacing, humor, solution, redirection/leading.)

PT: Umm... yeah I don't think I'll be scheduling...

DS: Ok, that's not a problem. We're always looking to find out how we can do better... do you mind if I ask why you don't want to schedule at this time?

(Again, you're probably being blown off, but it's more gentle and this person seems more undecided about booking, maybe even a little ashamed to have taken you up on a free or inexpensive offer and not give you anything in return. Your question to them is disarming and will flush out the real objections if there are any OR let them off the hook nicely and relieve tension in your communications.)

PT: Well my {tooth} is hurting so let's start with that one.

DS: Definitely. Sorry to hear you're in pain, let's see what's the soonest we can have you come in. I have two spots tomorrow and one on {day}. Which day works best for you?

(Whenever possible give the choice between something and something, not between something and nothing. If you're not an expert at this yet please study the funneling section of this script book.)

PT: Haha! You guys showed me $10,000 worth of treatment after a free exam and you want me to just come in and get it done?

DS: Haha, I understand… that's a long-term plan though. Doesn't mean you have to get it all done at once or even all done… but we can definitely take care of _____ or the _____ just to get you started. Do you want to do something like that or what's the other option?

(Pacing and leading. They laugh, you laugh. They talk about the huge amount, you let them know you understand by acknowledging the extensive nature of their treatment plan. Then you give them choices and put the ball in their court.)

PT: Actually no. I just came in because the exam was free/cheap but I have no intention of scheduling.

DS: Not a problem, we understand some people do that. Are you working with another dentist, or should I check back with you in ____ days/months?

(This forces them to either disqualify themselves by working with someone else OR gives you permission to contact them again. If they say something other than what you asked, that's an open door for your next leading question. Funnel funnel funnel!)

PT: {anything else that you hear as an initial objection regarding money, schedule, customer satisfaction, insurance, etc.}

DS: {anything that relieves stress from their statement if needed, a concise explanation, and a question to redirect the communication back to them and keep control of the conversation}

(You want the patient to be in question answering mode for the most part. It is your job as the dental professional they trust {or are testing to see if they can trust} to lead the conversation in a way that creates good will and income for your practice. At the very least they should hang up with you and think: Well, IF I were going to the dentist… I'd go to THAT dentist.)

PT: Yeah, that would be great! I got so lost not knowing where to start with so much to do in my mouth…

DS: I know, it happens a lot! It's not a problem though, I can help you figure out what would be the most important right now, just so you can get started. Is anything hurting or uncomfortable right now?

('Nuff said… pacing, choices, redirection.)

Auditory learning

This script book is accompanied by a set of audio samples that can help your staff learn the proper delivery of these scripts. Similar to learning a song, a little repetition goes a long way!

The audio program portion will show you there is no right or wrong with the words your say, as long as the intent of your communication is directed where you need it. Want the audios? Email me:

Juan@Hypnodontist.com

Remember all sales are a transference of emotion. You and your team provide a service you consider valuable to your patients' well-being and it's your job to ensure your communication conveys that emotion.

The next step for you and your practice

IMPLEMENTATION

Dear Doctor:

Would you like help implementing this material and offering your patients the added value of Hypnodontics? Please contact the practitioner who presented this book to you.

NOTE: We offer and license these materials for hypnosis practitioners the world over to offer dental practices empowering new ways to grow as they learn the language of ethical influence.

However, each practitioner is a separate entity from Hypnodontist.com and acting on his/her own accord. We cannot accept responsibility for their performance or attest to their competence with the subject matter. We sincerely hope your association to the person who gave you this book will pay off handsomely in a win/win/win format.

This content cannot be sold or traded except by its original author, Juan P. Acosta from Hypnodontist.com and it's offered for educational purposes.

Enjoy your new skills!

It takes a village...

This book as well as the content I've created for Hypnodontist does not happen by itself, and it would likely not happen if I were left to my own devices.

Many people have contributed to the building of this book and the skills I needed to work in the field to be able to write it.

I always like to show my appreciation for those choose to invest their time, their most valuable resource, to enjoy and use the content I produce and most importantly to help me with the essential tasks of proof-reading, editing and reviewing my materials before they go public.

Too many people deserve a mention here and I am grateful for their investment of time and resources to help me get this work in your hands.

For the purpose of brevity I will stick to sending a big thank you to the major players on this particular project: Kelley T. Woods, Kevin Cole, and the biggest thank you of all to my good friend and amazingly skilled business partner, Dave Berman, who has invested countless hours being over-worked and under-paid from this and other Hypnodontist projects. This book is yours as it is mine.

Thank you, sincerely.

More praise for Hypnodontics

*"As clinical practitioners, understanding not just *what* to communicate to patients, but *how* to ethically influence them to experience greater comfort and satisfaction in your office, is key to building and sustaining a successful practice. What "Hypnodontics" offers is a great intro to the world of ethical influence in a clinical environment for dental professionals." **Kevin Cole C.Ht. Founder of Empowerment Quest International & The Las Vegas Hypnosis Center***

*"Even if you apply only one technique from Juan Acosta's book, you'll find dramatic improvements in your practice - but of course, you'll want to learn all the communication methods he teaches to truly transform your patients' experience of dentistry." **James Hazlerig, MA, CHP***

*"This is a practical book that belongs in every dental practice. In these pages you will find everyday language to produce extraordinary results. Hypnodontist has created the right words to use at the right time for each member of your team so you expand your practice in an elegant way." **Dan Paris, CHP***

*"Thanks Juan... Hypnodontics is very practical and to the point. I have many books and completed quite a few courses on hypnotism, however your book impressed me with its practicality." **Zahid Ansari, B.E , BAMS, C.Ht.***

"Hypnodontics does a great job of illustrating how dentists can effectively apply the language of ethical influence to help produce more comfortable patients and more profitable treatment plans. From case presentation, to call handling, to helping anxious or fearful patients achieve optimal oral health, your entire team will be well-served by reading this book. Hypnodontics by Juan P. Acosta, CHP, is a must-read for any dentist looking to better serve their patients while simultaneously boosting their bottom line." **Chris Barnard, Managing Partner, Social Dental Network**

"Juan Acosta's book is packed full of simple ways to dramatically improve your dental practice. You can get started today towards increasing your patients' comfort and compliance by utilizing these transformative techniques." **Katie Sandlin, CCH, MS**

"Coming from one of those freaked out dental patients, I think this book deserves to be at every dentist's office and I wish it were! My dentist will be getting a copy... ;)" **Trish Pavlecich, Writer, Soon-to-be ex-dental phobic**

No more fear, your Hypnodontist is here.

Hypnodontist.com